FIGHT

OF

FAITH

JAMES MOODY

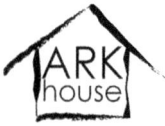

Ark House Press
PO Box 1722, Port Orchard, WA 98366 USA
PO Box 1321, Mona Vale NSW 1660 Australia
PO Box 318 334, West Harbour, Auckland 0661 New Zealand
arkhousepress.com

Cataloguing in Publication Data:
Title: Fight of Faith
ISBN: 978-0-6488873-5-5 (pbk)
Subjects: Faith; Christian Living;
Other Authors/Contributors: Moody, James

Design by initiateagency.com

■ ACKNOWLEDGEMENTS

To my mum and dad for fighting my battles with me; all those that uttered prayers my way covering me with a blanket of prayer; and to God who is my strength.

■ FOREWORD
Corey Turner

I first met James Moody many years ago when he reached out to me and asked me to be his mentor. What a privilege to be asked to speak into somebody else's life. Whilst it's not always possible to fulfil every request for coaching or mentoring, there was a prompting of the Spirit in my heart, that I should make myself available and meet up with James.

As I chatted with him in our first meeting, it became very clear that he was passionate about Jesus, hungry to learn and very focused on discovering and fulfilling his calling. What was also apparent was that he had a maturity about him, beyond his years, that had been developed in the crucible of pain. His outlook on life and faith in Jesus had been forged in a firestorm of circumstances that required James to cling to Jesus for survival.

James' book 'Fight of Faith' is the story of James' battle against cancer and more importantly his journey into finding faith in Jesus Christ as the Son of God. As James shares his story across each page, you will discover, that God is as intimately involved in the details of your life as he was involved in James' life. You'll be encouraged by the truth that God is as interested in the minutia of your daily existence as much as he is interested in the broad brushstrokes of your deepest pain and wildest adventure.

This book has been a long time coming and much work has been invested into it. James doesn't write as if he is a spectator of someone else's testimony. He writes from the depths of his own journey which gives his message such credibility. As you read each page, you'll encounter key themes like grace, faith, perseverance and humility. All of these are much needed qualities for each of our lives.

I know that as you read 'Fight of Faith', you will be inspired and challenged to not only fight your own battles with grace and courage but you will discover that true life and God's peace is ultimately found in a personal and intimate faith in Christ.

Corey Turner is the Senior Pastor of Neuma Church, a multi-location church, birthed in revival 100 years ago with a rich heritage in church planting and global mission. He is a recognised prophetic voice across the wider body of Christ and has authored several books. He has a Bachelor of Ministry from Tabor College and resides in Melbourne, Australia with his wife Simone and three amazing kids, Chelsea, Zack and Joshua.

██████ PROLOGUE

God.

The word 'God' brings so many differing thoughts, emotions, questions and notions. It is possibly the heaviest connoted word we have in our language. It invokes meaning in what we have seen, heard, learnt and been taught when it comes to God. The reality is, we all have questions when it comes to God. It is whether we act on those questions to find out more, ignore it because it is not a priority, or simply dismiss it as nothing. I know I certainly had questions and I still do, despite what I have discovered for myself so far on my journey. Some questions may be broad. "Is there a God?"; "Is God real?"; "Is there more than one god?"; "What does God do?" Or more specific: "Does God care about me?"; "What is a characteristic of God?" and so on. It is like trying to discover information about another human being that has been spoken about, taught about, assumed about, only that there is conflicting information and embellished stories through the differing beliefs, perspectives and lived experiences. Where do we start?

I am attempting to begin by throwing my little pebble into this mountain of rocks and welcome you to my journey of discovering God. This is my personal story of how God has shaped my life through experiences, battles, trials, direction, preconceived notions and dialogue so far.

Wisdom.

This sets the stage for me to open my Bible to the book of James… naturally, going to my namesake. In James 1:5, this passage resonates with my story:

> *"If any of you lacks wisdom, you should ask God, who gives generously to all without finding fault and it will be given to you."*

I understand wisdom to be the very substance of knowing and applying said knowledge into our lives. Wisdom is the highest understanding we can receive from God (when he is known as above everything else in our lives) and this understanding includes faith, strength, stamina, clarity, direction and so on. This gold nugget tells me that whatever I am lacking, whether it is wisdom, or something to help me draw closer to God such as faith, I can simply ask God and he will give it to me.

Trials.

There is, however, a prerequisite here that I understand. The verses prior to it in James 1:2-4 talks about trials.

> *"Consider it pure joy, my brothers and sisters, whenever you face trials of many kinds, because you know that the testing of your faith produces perseverance. Let perseverance finish its work so that you may be mature and complete, not lacking anything"*

God will use trials to sharpen the very things I ask for which I lack. I cannot simply become adept at a specific skill without trying to learn.

I need to go through the act of learning, practising, applying and mastering. In the same way, through the challenges of life, and something I ask God to help me with; I can be sharpened and matured in the areas I need to draw closer to God and to help me navigate this grand journey called life.

This is the beauty of this piece found in the book of James. All of us go through challenges in life, all go through peaks and troughs. All of us have plateaus, which creates the many opportunities for God to sharpen us. We often ignore it. God speaks to us in many ways and forms. Too often, as humans, we can throw our arms up at God, dismayed because God has not verbally spoken to us. Chances are he has, but we miss the small voice in the loud wind. We are preoccupied with distractions, disruptions and perhaps disobedience. I know that God has spoken to you, I know God has called out to you, but it is the matter of whether you heard it or not; whether the voice was given an ear to listen to or stifled, whether you were aware of it or not. What is God trying to share with you today?

Jigsaw.

Looking back on this whole situation, how it all unfolded was like fitting a jigsaw puzzle together. As my family and I join the pieces together, we marvel at the way God works everything out. He masterfully weaves everything together to make sure it all works into His favour. God's impeccable timing is not to be underestimated. God's continuous blessings throughout the trials allowed provision and support for my journey. God's teachings are profound and have never left my heart and never will. God's ability to impact millions through one's fight is to never be undermined. God's hand over my life was so strong that the situation I faced looked like a mere problem and one easy to overcome.

I want to share as much as I can in this book because I want to help increase an awareness of how God could be dealing with your situation. There are so many blessings in disguise that come our way that we often forget to stop and think about these small things. It's time to slow down, smell the roses and listen to God so we can become far more aware of God's impact in our lives, how He is dealing with our circumstances and what He wants us to do.

The supreme argument for God is not through theology or intellectual debates, but through experiencing the transformative and restorative power of God. This is my story of how I discovered God as a friend who wants to walk with me in my life and every day. Here we go!

■■■■■■ START.

Household.

I was born and raised in a loving, stable, strong Christian household. I love my parents for their unconditional love for me and their unwavering conviction in God. They brought me up in an environment of Christian values and morals, a house filled with love and salted with grace.

Dad always had a strong, authoritative presence. He brooded over me like a superman, ready to catch me if I was ever in danger. He had a strong heart of love that advocated for my development and growth in my life. His strength appeared in many forms and I am so thankful for the strong arm that lifted me up continuously as I grappled with the ropes of life. As a child, I could never beat Dad when it came to defying him. I was going through a stage of growing up as a young teenager where you begin to go through changes physically, mentally and emotionally. You soon learn where the boundaries are. I was becoming selfish, rude and showing no grace to the people around me. Dad took away all my privileges—phone, laptop, television—to the point that I was dwelling only in my anger, frustration and scorn. This is the most defining season that taught me true love, real kindness and sincere courtesy is always the way to go when it comes to navigating life. Dad's mandate that he preaches all the time is *you always face the consequences of your actions. Healthy decisions reap healthy results; unhealthy decisions reap unhealthy consequences.* This mandate shapes how I live my life; with a mindfulness of others and an understanding that everything I do has a result, so everything I do is my responsibility.

Mum was nurtured in a Christian household too, with my grandparents being pastors of a prolific church movement. Everything she put her hand to was always of love, care, kindness, effort and intention. Her actions have taught me how to empathize, care and love for others in a way others feel seen, heard, known and loved.

My older sister, Jess, is a person who has paved the way beyond me as the senior sibling and constantly challenges my thoughts, ideas and notions of my own experiences. It is another layer that builds understanding, awareness and a greater perspective beyond my own sense of self. Having this great family dynamic assisted my development in such a healthy way. It allowed me to grow with a strong sense of morality, understanding that great love encompasses all and that said, great love is found from God, with a growing understanding that there are so many different views of God. I was beginning to critically analyse everything that was taught about God; the little things that didn't add up in my own feeble mind.

Doubt.

With this critical mindset, I befriended a person who leeches onto this kind of thinking: Doubt. Doubt embraced me with a big side shoulder hug and promised me that we were going to go on a great journey. Doubt rushed in without my consent and I, unknowingly, entered a wrestling match with God. I was walking with Doubt everywhere I went. Before I knew it, his words were influencing my way of thinking. Everything he says gnaws at you. It is evident in your mind as you think, analyse, wonder and think again sceptically. Doubt in self, doubt in others, doubt in God. With Doubt, he created a sense of insecurity in myself: how I looked, how I acted and how I thought. Doubt pushed me to try a fit in the norm of school, teenage years, and being a boy at the expense of changing who I am.

Comfortable.

Something always felt a little different. I had another great friend whom I relied on heavily. His name was Comfortable. He always brought a sense of ease into my life. Comfortable indulges in the fact I have good opportunities and access that come down my way. I live a decent and comfortable lifestyle. Good family, good school, good church, good health and a good lifestyle. Nothing more, nothing less. Comfortable brought great balance with my friendship with Doubt. He is the encourager while Doubt taught me to be reasonable and sceptical. Doubt and Comfortable took their roles as my great advisors for life.

There is an acquaintance, however, that I could never put away or get rid of. He is a person of so many different reputations. I heard different stories, but never really took the chance to know him. Deep inside, I really wanted to know the true representation and character of who he is, but I feared what Doubt and Comfortable would think of me if I tried. This acquaintance is God.

I was not satisfied with my only two friends, Doubt and Comfortable. A belief within me began stirring; that there is more to what I was seeing and living. God always had a smile on his face. I felt there was something different about him, but I could not put my finger on it. I did not know him close enough. I crave to have more encounters with him because of all the stories I had heard about him. God was helping people discover their identity, purpose and love. I do not know how, but it was happening. Doubt jumped on my back and applied strong pressure on my insecurity. I was never secure. I was never good enough. Comfortable raised his arm on my shoulder and gave me a friendly reminder that I have it good; I do not need to find anything better. I continued living the same way, but something was different. There was a spiritual craving within my soul to have a real encounter with God. This craving was burning within me because it was in direct contrast of Doubt and Comfortable.

I was surrounded by the notion and concept of God, through my parent's beliefs, the teachings and culture of the church, which I attended weekly. It was part of my life. I built relationships with people who believed in God. There was a disconnect in what I knew and heard about God and what I perceived to be true about God in my own life. I never saw God do the very things that people have said that he has done. My heart burned for what my ears were hearing to be true, but Doubt continued to over-process and poke holes in the beliefs that were trying to establish in my mind and heart. I wanted to have this unwavering belief that God is legitimate and have a concrete reason to believe it, to see something that God does and realise what all the fuss is about. I decided to do something new: I began praying for my own encounter with God that would give me a reason to believe he was real and to become close to him. I wanted the opportunity to say *God is real* and show others why ever so clearly because of my own lived experience and relationship with God. I craved this revelation. I wanted a new friend to give me a new outlook on life; to help me be secure, at peace, purposeful and with direction. I wanted more! In the meantime, Doubt continued to remind me of what I lacked as I rested in the warm arms of Comfortable.

Disconnect.

I feel for God. Doubt has brought so much hindrance to people trying to get to know him. Some people attend church for years and abide by his teachings, yet Doubt creates that strong hesitancy when it comes to wanting to know God as a friend, who wants to share the experiences in your life. Doubt makes you feel insecure by stating that God is closer to other people than you; that God has personal experiences with others that you cannot relate to. Doubt attempts to make your lack of worthiness obvious to you so you cannot be with God. Doubt causes you to question whether God really is all that he is. You might grow up near God and hear about God, but what you have experienced in your life causes you to truly embrace Doubt's words. This is the great disconnect. The gap that makes you either turn away because it seems too great for you to overcome, or it makes you hungry for God because you know there is more to it.

I grew up hearing stories of peoples' personal battles and how they beat drugs, or grew up in a broken home and met God, who revolutionises their lives. For me, this was enhancing my relationship with Doubt. Doubt convinced me that logically, it came down to two points: they are lying and it merely happened through coincidence, or I simply had not had an experience with God yet. I wanted God to revolutionize my life somehow: that I could come out of a bad situation victorious through God and be an inspiration for others. This became my deep, embedded-in-my-heart prayer: to face a tough situation, get to know God and overcome it with him. I prayed this prayer subconsciously, not knowing what I really was wishing for. Comfortable shied his eyes away in horror at the thought of this prayer and Doubt grumbled at my attempts to undermine him.

Encounter.

In the year 2006, the craving of wanting more created a significant moment at a Christian conference I attended yearly. It was a fun routine trip every year, until one year, the ordinary conference became a relevant conference. The conference was always bustling with people who were so expectant for God to speak to them. This always fuelled my scepticism when I never really heard God speak to me. I chose to enrol in the Brotherhood class, which Dad encouraged me to be a part of. Dad shared that it was perfect for men my age. It was a class where all boys got together, talked about issues and topics that came up in the lives of boys growing up. That year, the theme was 'dreams'. When I first heard it, I thought to myself, *I already have this covered. I want to be a football player!* Like most young boys at a young age, this was pretty much the norm. It's amazing how we think we already know everything at twelve years old! As the facilitators spoke more about the topic on dreams, I started to realise that they were talking about something different, bigger and better. I could not quite grasp what it was. My spirit was beginning to twitch and squirm. As my spirit was being stirred, I approached the leader who led the brotherhood elective. I do not mess around, so I blurted out to him, "I don't have a dream," to which he replied, "Yes, you do, you can ask God for it." It all seemed too easy to me. He sat me down next to him and he laid his hand on my shoulder and prayed to God for him to deliver my dream and bring breakthrough into my life. We left it at that. Nothing was different, just an exchange of a simple question and answer.

At the night show of the conference, there was a UK Christian band performing. I was shouting out the lyrics to their songs at the top of my lungs, enjoying myself with a friend. As I was engaging with the songs, a moment occurred which was very strange. My lips were moving to the words of the songs, but within an instant and momentarily, different words came out of my mouth. The specific words that came out were *my dream is to have a life-inspiring story that will change people's lives.* Then my voice reverted to the lyrics I was singing and soon after, I stopped in silence as the moment hit me. I just had an experience with a friend called God. I quickly sprinted out of the auditorium and gleefully texted my mother what had just happened. I was in awe and amazed at my first encounter. I stood there, stunned. The leader in the brotherhood class was indeed correct! All I had to do was approach God and ask. This was my first significant moment with my friend, God. The stories about God were beginning to look true.

Pledged.

Shortly after my encounter with God, I was still dealing with my friends, Doubt and Comfortable. Old habits remained; my normal lifestyle continued. Although my spirit and sense of self was different, as I knew I ought to pursue more, I did not know how. A pastor in his sixties shared of his friendship with God in front of the assembly of people. He developed a healing ministry. I set out a challenge for God with one of my biggest driving forces for Doubt: my deafness. As I was born, I was diagnosed with a severe hearing loss. I wore hearing aids from a baby to this day to assist my hearing. It was my biggest obstacle for when it came to knowing God because it influenced my relationship with doubt. I am grateful that I could hear with the assistance of hearing aids, but part of me always wanted to be hearing and even more, have a story of being dramatically healed. As a young child, I usually felt embarrassed to be deaf, especially when people would rudely point to my ears and shout '*What's that in your ear?*' It made me feel alienated, different from the rest. I was still coming to grips with my identity and sense of self. I felt like I missed out on things. Every time I heard people saying *God can heal you.* I always wondered if that was true because why I was still deaf? I would answer the call when people asked, *is there anyone that needs healing?* They would pray for me and nothing would happen, causing my faith to take a huge hit and decrease.

Other people would answer the call and be healed from blindness, cancer, limps, back problems, paralysis and every other need they could heal. This further propelled me to become a sceptic. I can relate to the story of *Doubting Thomas* in John 20:24-29, who refuses to believe that Jesus was alive, until he saw him with his very own eyes and touched him with his very own hands. In this situation again, challenging God to heal me, I swallowed my pride and walk up to the front as the pastor called up people for healing. I shared with him my deafness and he began praying over my ears. Nothing changed. He tried a few more times and same result. My spirit was still stirred and I was deep in thought, racking my brain, attempting to make sense of all this. I could not keep doing the same thing and expect different results. Something has to change or work for me. The pastor wrapped up the healing proceedings and shared that beyond all the miracles, God simply wants us to be with him. His focus is more on spiritual healing than physical. The pastor urged us to respond to that call and be his friend. *Maybe that's what I ought to do?* I followed the promptings of my spirit. I began to bargain with God *'I'm going to give you a chance. I am going to give my life to you and you can do what you want with it. If nothing has changed in a few years, then I will move on, knowing I tried and it did not work out. This is your chance to help me build a relationship with you.'* In that moment, I pledged to walk with God. I did not know what to expect, but I knew I wanted to know more about God.

Ripeness.

In 2008, two years after my first encounter with God and choosing to walk with God as a friend, despite my relationships with Doubt and Comfortable, there was a woman at my church, Roxy, who had a fierce passion that was developed from her relationship with God. She continually taught people her own revelations from walking with God. God introduced her to me to help initiate a rapid growth in my relationship with him. A Sunday rolled around and Roxy pulled me aside with my good friend, Nat, to assist her. Roxy began to speak over my life and said, *'You are ripe. You are at that age where God wants to take you on a great journey, teach you and strengthen your spirit. You are ripe for the taking, no matter what people say to you. You and only you need to believe it yourself and take it with both hands. You are ripe!'*

I absorbed these words, nodding away. Roxy and Nat prayed over me with great passion and that was the end. I walked away, not realising the power of these words and the notion that Roxy had prophesised over my life. From the very next day, God unleashed a powerful spiritual growth in my life. God poured out His wisdom into my life, I began writing dozens of messages about certain topics, establishing my passion of learning, reading and writing. I was seeing things in a different way. God revealed to me how to hear his voice, as well as the power of prayer. I was feeling like I gained VIP access to God. I was the privileged friend who was invited to witness this wondrous environment that God walks in daily. As part of the growth, I discovered a passion that God revealed to me. I asked my pastor for an opportunity to share something to a small group of friends at my youth. Pastor Enzo gave me the okay and told me I had fifteen minutes coming up that next Friday. I diligently wrote down what I wanted at the meeting. I absolutely revel in the passion and joy of preaching. I spoke on God's purpose and having the courage to achieve it. While preaching, it became an incredible moment because something clicked for me. My spirit came alive. Like a person who nails a song at a concert for the first time, one who auditions for a role in a theatre, one who picks up a basketball and knows that this is what they want to do for the rest of their lives, I knew I want to preach for the rest of my life. It was electric; passion and purpose, colliding together, creating the most beautiful sense of joy. Another friend of God, who became my mentor, explained that you can tell what God purposes you for when you're doing something intuitively and it clicks and resonates with your spirit. God does not entrust us with passions, talents, gifts and expect us not to utilize them. I discovered my purpose. God was enjoying our relationship as it deepened and I was saturated by his presence. I was enjoying it, being a privileged friend of God. The stories of God were being proven true at every corner of our journey.

Aftermath.

Just like any relationship, it certainly was not all smooth sailing. I was engulfed in the presence of God, but there were things I still needed to work on. The bigger challenges followed. After a few months of rapid spiritual growth, after preaching, after learning the ways of God and developing as a Christian, it all came to a sudden halt. God became distant once again. God did not seem to be around anymore. It completely came as a surprise and I did not expect it. I was not prepared in the dealings of it. I tried to recapture that burning desire and everything I felt during those crazy months, but nothing worked. I could not quite grasp what was happening. Relationship difficulties bear emotional turmoil.

In panic, I ran to my old friend, Comfortable, for warmth and security. Doubt heard how I was feeling and came back to me with an *I told you so*. I went back to old habits and my old lifestyle. Being with God in that season was like a bond that completely changes your world and nothing is the same again, but life still moves forward, somehow with or without. As I attempted to recapture the feeling I had when God was with me, I gave up and reverted back to my old ways. I did not seek God, pray, meditate or worship him. I did not chase him because the 'feeling' and drive was not there. Doubt came back with more ammunition to instil more scepticism in my life and relationship with God. The only thing that kept me believing was all the revelations I had received from God.

Relationship Dynamic.

This was a learning curve for me as I realised I could not base my lifestyle and relationships on emotions. There are times in your life when God pulls away to see how you will respond. There are times in your life when friends pull away to see if you will chase after them. There are times when your significant other pulls away to see if you notice because if you love them, you will. The real challenge from God was after everything he did for me, will I seek him and continue to walk on the small path that God has set out for me, or will I revert to my old ways and walk away from him? This is the true measuring stick of your faith and belief in God. If you truly trust him, you will trust him when he's there and when he *seems* to be invisible. This is when the depth of your love and relationship with God is revealed. The good thing about relationships is that they can develop further. If you disappoint yourself when God first 'disappears' by turning back, it is not the end of the world. We need to chase God once again, get things right with him and learn from the experience so that God can develop our relationship and increase our faith and trust in him.

Story-Teller.

I disappointed myself with the action of turning away and not chasing after God, despite the understanding I developed in my relationship with God. God decided to give me an opportunity to be passionate once again. Out of routine, I attended church every Friday and Sunday for youth services and church services respectively. A guest speaker came one Friday with an uncommon message to share, one that I did not believe would be as significant as it came to be later. The speaker shared his passion of telling stories. Storytelling is an art that needs to be encouraged. I am shocking at storytelling. I get to the punch line too quickly that nobody is laughing or intrigued because my story is under-developed in details. The speaker makes a statement that rings through my brain: *everybody has a story to tell!* My imaginative fist went up ready to fight. I did not have a story to tell. I was too comfortable and too insecure. He shared that everyone has a personal, unique story to tell, which can impact others. I could not shake the feeling that my story did not compare in measurement of impact to those stories of people overcoming drugs, sickness, abuse, loneliness, or brokenness. These were the stories that captivate, inspire and challenge others to overcome their own situation. I began to get frustrated because this message was hitting a personal spot and I did not know why. I continued to crave for a great story to tell. I cried out to God that moment and ranted on how I lived a comfortable life with a good family, friends, education and health. I questioned how I can reach out to these people with a story to tell. How am I going to be inspiration for others, when quite frankly, I do not inspire myself?

God took a seat next to me in silence and I became aware of his presence. God waited for me to calm down so I could be ready to listen. '*Do you remember the dream I gave you?*' he asked me. As clear as anything, the words come back to mind, '*to have a life-inspiring story that will change people's lives*'. Never have I felt so far from a dream.

'*Trust me that I will never fail to deliver what I have promised you. This message is for you to be reminded of what I want to give you. Chase after me, walk with me and I will give all this to you. Be ready: I am going to teach you. I am going to fast track your development so that you can be ready when I call you. I am going to overload you with understanding and knowledge! Just keep persisting with me no matter what.*'

God really asked a lot from me that day; but it was the slap in the face I needed. I was demanding God to give me something while I was resting on my laurels, not really caring about pursuing Him. Imagine asking a husband or wife to do something for you when you have not even acknowledged their presence for weeks! The very next day, God began to move in the exact fashion he promised me he would. There are many events that I can touch on where I can see God progressively building up my relationship with Him; working in me with so that he could work through me. There are the events and areas in your life where you know God touched you and it brought a breath of fresh air in your spirit. It is these events that reveal God's love for us and allows us to catch a glimpse of God. I pray that you hold onto these revelations and do not forget them, especially when you are in a challenging season. Allow it to propel you deeper into God's presence and love. In this season, I simply needed to pursue as I held what God revealed to me close to my heart. What I did not know was my health started to deteriorate that day.

Aromas.

In June 2009, I was gifted an opportunity to work in a retail store for a week for experience to increase my chances of gaining employment later in life. It was a big chain store that sold many home ware and living items. My job was to restock everything that the management gaves me; from kitchenware, to bed sheets, to clothes. Half way through the week, I got asked to stock up the aromatic candles on the shelves. As I looked at them, there was a plethora of aromas: lavender, rose, vanilla, spice and everything else I can think of. Being slightly OCD when it comes to organising myself and wanting everything to be in its rightful place, I took it upon myself to rearrange all the candles so that each scent was placed together. I spent the next hour foolishly sorting out the mammoth scented candles. My nose was amid the aromas. Slowly, the aromas collectively built up into a powerful cloud that began to move towards my nose, my mouth breathing in copious amounts. It was like I was eating soap. I pushed through to ensure I was finishing the task I set out to do. My throat was clogging up and I could not work out what the smell was anymore as it was getting too much. I completed the task and walked away from it, trying to recover with a little bit of fresh air. Next thing I know, I was sick and weak. I never came back for the rest of the week because my body was in agony, weak and weary. I spent the next few days living in my bed with a horrible cold, sore throat, throbbing headache, no energy and no appetite. Recovering from the sickness, I brushed it off as a general flu and thought nothing of it anymore.

Basketball.

I play basketball weekly and it is a passion of mine. It is my favourite way of being immersed in something exciting that enables me to enjoy what is happening now and forget what is happening around me. It is a sport that teaches me how to challenge myself to be better and how to work with the people around me, in the face of an opposition. I am generally fit and have an ability to run out games well, despite how much energy I expend throughout. After being sick, I noticed in basketball each week I played that I seemed to have less stamina, less petrol in the tank to finish off games. I was half way through a game and I was breathing heavily, even though I was not doing too much beyond my capacity. *I've really got to start eating healthier before games. Those big, juicy burgers are not ideal beforehand.* I assure myself that it is a dietary thing. I continued to push myself and finish off the games, but I felt that I was not doing so within the best of my ability because of fatigue. It was frustrating, not being able to do something as well as you usually do, or better.

Flu.

September 2009. Three months after my first flu from the aromatic candles, I get very sick again with the exact same symptoms, except no aroma candles. That was deducted from the equation. Again, I spent the next few days living in my bed with a horrible cold, sore throat, throbbing headache, no energy and no appetite. It was frustrating having to put your life on hold for a whole week because you have been knocked out by something that affects you physically. To have to go through it twice in the space of four months was worse and amplified the frustration. One week passed by and I could move around. One key difference remained:

even though I felt better, I did not have the same energy or vibrancy that I normally carried. As a person who played sports competitively, I could not even jog ten metres without gasping for breath. My face was pale. Mum would always comment *'You are white as a ghost!'* Thanks for the compliment! My energy became something that I needed to preserve and only expend if I needed to. It was like a person with a shortage of money: they need to pick and choose what they want to invest in. Do they choose to take that offer of lunch with someone for enjoyment, or do they choose to say no, to possibly pay for petrol for a few days? As a teenager, I wanted to live my life having fun and enjoying myself with others. I chose to push myself, muster up the efforts to be in other people's company, but it was not easy. I summoned the strength to go to a camp and pretended that everything was okay. My lack of energy acted as an obstacle as I needed lots of sleep and rest to keep up with the daily activities. I continually retreated privately to catch my breath and recover my energy. It became a constant cycle. Do, then rest, and repeat. I jumped in the activities because I do not want to miss out. I would do my hardest to complete the objective, then whenever I got the chance, I would stop, breathe and do it over again.

Iron Levels.

No one really picked up at that point that I was unwell or something was up because I was doing a good job concealing my weaknesses and vulnerabilities through enthusiasm and participation. My family and I, however, knew something was not right. I complained of having little energy and not feeling like my normal self. We scheduled an appointment with my family doctor. He gave me a blood test and checked out the results. The doctor amused himself with the results a few times over.

He could not quite analyse the results properly with what he had. *'The iron levels are too high, but the red blood cell count is too low. I am not sure why this is occurring.'* I have my first details gathered. Too high iron, low blood levels. Got it. Doc referred me to the Children's Ward at Monash Hospital and we proceeded further there. Here was a crazy thought: my mother suggested I take iron tablets before I got my check-up, as my symptoms may be a result of low iron. If I had taken iron tablets, not realizing I had high iron levels, there would have been devastating results, as I would have 'overdosed' on iron and deceased. Thank God I did not take any because I wanted to be sure of what was going on!

Monash.

Eventually, the issue was discovered that my iron was not converting into blood cells as quickly as it should be, resulting in high iron levels. My body's balance was out of whack. Over the few months at Monash, I was playing a waiting game. It was frustrating. Not being able to find out what the issue was, therefore, not being able to move forward towards an outcome. It was like driving a car around a roundabout continuously; no exit or destination in sight. I am normally driven by progress and results, but this was the opposite side of the spectrum. I had repeated bone marrow biopsies, which is an examination of the tissue removed from my bone marrow to discover the cause or extent of a disease. The doctors still struggled to work out why my blood results were revealing what they revealed. The initial thought is that it was a virus that has affected my system. They decide that I ought to get blood donations to boost up my low blood count and hopefully, it would kick start my bone marrow function back up to speed. Over the course of three months, fortnightly, I had to go to the hospital to receive blood donations. Two bags of blood took six hours to transfer into my body. I was fortunate enough to be able to finish school early on Wednesdays, but unfortunate that I had to spend my free afternoons in the hospital. Each fortnight, for the six hours, I would fill my time with homework, movies and sleeping. After another biopsy and more blood tests, my blood levels continued to decrease back to the same amount. Even worse, other figures in my results dropped even more. Nothing was stemming the flow and I could not maintain the blood in my system. This was a cause for concern.

God's Request

With everything out of my control, my blood levels dropping, I took it to God. I asked God to do something, anything. Heal me. God shared that he had other ideas. God imparted his advice: *'Why don't you tell the people around you what is wrong with your blood system so that they are aware of the problem and then I will heal you? That way you can glorify my name. They can know that the stories about me are true, through you.'* It sounded like a simple request, although I have never been a person who openly speaks about my personal life at school. I usually share when I am asked to do so; that way I am not feeling like I am burdening other people with my problems. It may have been a confidence thing: what if they do not care? I brush off the request and continue my routine of going to school, hospital every fortnight, and my usual activities. No one outside my family really knew what was going on. The only moments that people may have picked up something was when I would be lacking energy and people asked if I was okay, because I am not my usual vibrant self. I always responded by sharing that I was okay, just tired. As I had a reputation of having an enjoyable, optimistic spirit, it came as a shock to people when they saw me trying to carry myself along, struggling to keep up with the demands of school. As the news eventually came out later, some people were surprised when they heard that I was going through health problems because I was actively doing school and sports. People did not realise that when I got home, I would crash and nap daily. Not many people knew what was going on as I was enduring the initial battle. If they did, they did not know much about it.

Situations.

Having to push myself through my schedule at school, without many people knowing, paints a valuable lesson that I have carried with me onwards. It is amazing how much we do not know when it comes to what others are facing in their everyday lives. We do not know what fights people are battling daily and going through. It revealed to me that every single person is facing a personal situation, whether it is physical, emotional, mental, spiritual, situational, or addictions. I question what would happen if people began to open up a little bit, show a little more vulnerability and transparency? It is humbling when people share with me a personal issue because I discover that I am not alone, and neither are they. It puts it into perspective that the world does not revolve around me and my own situations. It enables me to reach out and provide a means of support and love they may need, despite what I am going through. It creates influence as I support and encourage another person who has allowed themselves to be vulnerable and confide in me. What would happen if we had the boldness and courage to open up a little bit more with others who we trust?

Overdrive.

January 2010. Dr Downie decides that before my next biopsy, we should try a long shot. It is the 'Hail Mary' of blood donations. He decides that we should pump a mammoth amount of blood into my system with the hope that the Bone Marrow will miraculously respond positively. It seems ridiculous, does it not? That's usually what happens when you have scoured all areas and have nothing to lose. Crazier things have happened. With a sense of optimism, I agree to it. Instead of two blood bags. I had four bags of blood pushed into my system at a rapid rate. The doctors were a little too giddy for my confidence. I began hoping that maybe something indeed could happen. The Hail Mary play was thrown. I was eagerly waiting to see if it would result in a touchdown. Over the course of the fortnight, my family monitored my progress. I was constantly probed with questions: *how are you feeling? Do you feel any different? Do you feel better? Any changes?* I could not answer any questions because it was too early to tell. I went back in for a blood test to see if anything had changed. The same result showed. I lost all the blood in my system back to the same level it usually dropped to, despite the great amount I had pumped in. Defeat overcame me. The ball spilled out of the hands and no touchdown resulted. We lost the game for that moment. In my moment of defeat, God decided to move onto the next game, since I did not carry out his request to speak out about my illness.

Optimism

February 2010. After the failure of the bulk blood donation attempt, I was turned in to have another Bone Marrow biopsy to see if anything else had developed, especially with the fact that my blood results were coming out worse. It became routine to me. I went in apathetically. There was no sense of expectation, no desire to pray and believe. I went in and out and awaited the results, believing that nothing was to be different. The next day I was called in for the appointment. Sitting down, I was defeated. Mum came in with a smile and a tinge of enthusiasm. *'I just saw Dr Peter. He's excited to see you. Apparently, they have some news.'* I perk up slightly. This ambiguity compels some curiosity from me. I rack my brain, trying to figure out what it may be. Whatever it is, is it a quick fix? Is it good news? Am I better? Optimism rose in my spirit at the thought of having an answer. The wait started to feel a little too long as my curiosity got ahead of itself.

Answer

Dr Peter greeted me with the trademark big grin and shook my hand. He motioned me to enter the room with him. I glanced around and there were five chairs. A strong, silent tension filled the room. I could not work out if it was a sense of optimism or seriousness that filled the atmosphere of the room. I sat down on one of the chairs, Mum taking her seat next to me. Dr Peter sat in front of me. His medical team entered: my nurse, Katy, and my health consultant took their seats next to Dr Peter. We all looked at each other, no words spoken, wondering how to begin the motions. This was the moment that the last two years of my life had been building up to. All the numerous blood donations, biopsies, appointments, illnesses, failures; all accumulated to work out the next step.

Dr Peter sliced the tension with a gentle tone as he began speaking. Dr Peter thoroughly ran through my medical history to paint the canvas of the journey so far. He pinpointed all the different avenues that they tried to jumpstart my Bone Marrow system to help me produce quality blood cells. He started sharing that my Bone Marrow had been struggling to produce for a while and my blood components were slowly decreasing in quality. He had my full attention. I had no idea where he was going to finish with this. Was he giving me a death sentence? Had he explored every avenue for no avail? I started to feel nervous, but he had my full focus. Dr Peter stated that it was time to act and that they had found an answer.

Then the punchline came. *You are diagnosed with a form of cancer. Myelodysplastic Syndrome (MDS).*

Dr Peter elaborated further. It is a disorder that affects normal blood cell production in the bone marrow. The bone marrow was currently producing abnormal, immature blood cells that did not help me function well. It is referred to as a pre-leukemic disorder. It was the very reason why my blood was not giving me the necessary nutrients my body needed to perform. I nod my head, dazed. Dr Peter continues, *'you will need a bone marrow transplant.'*

I breathed slowly, relief overcoming me. I felt no feelings of rage or sadness, just relief. I finally had an answer. It did come in the form of having a cancerous disease, but I had an answer; I had something concrete to help me move forward in this ordeal. This sickness slowly developed; it was not sudden, to the point that I wanted to simply move onwards. My family and I knew something was wrong and after the arduous journey of health appointments, we had an answer. I still did not fully comprehend the diagnosis. I did not understand what lay ahead for me because it was uncharted territory. Relief was met with nerves. What was next? My health consultant attempted to bring comfort to me. *'This is not your fault. It is pure bad luck'.* She mentions the reasons being that I do not smoke, drink, have bad fitness or diet.

Pure bad luck. Such comforting words when your life changes course and you have no control over it. *Pure bad luck.* When you now have to go through a Bone Marrow Transplant, which potentially has a lifetime of adverse side-affects. *Pure bad luck.* Now I have to put my education and aspirations on hold in order to focus on my health. *Pure bad luck.* Especially that ninety percent of people diagnosed with this disorder are over sixty-five years old in age. *Pure bad luck.* Since I did nothing to cause this sickness, it happened by natural causes of my body. *Pure bad luck.*

Nothing was making sense anymore. How was I supposed to process this news? Thoughts ran through my mind as nothing was clear. I did not know where to start. I had no control in helping myself get better. It was not my fault, nor did I have anything within my power to fix it. I walked to the one person that could do something about it. That set up everything for the dominos to fall.

Surrender.

With this new life news, I approached God. I felt numb, lacking clarity. Powerless. Something was stirring in my spirit, propelling me to go and converse with God. I humbled myself in his presence, laying myself at his feet as I attempted to gather my thoughts. There was a lightness in the air. It felt like I was in a different dimension with God, just me and him. I held the situation in my hands and handed it over to him. I look at God and instantly know what I need to do. It was mutual. I opened my mouth and spoke.

'God, I cannot do anything about this situation. If I could, I would fix it right now. The best thing I can do is give the situation to you and leave it in your hands. Take it! In the Bible, you promise to deliver the best outcome in

even the worst of circumstances if we trust and have faith in you. I promise that I will do so, especially when things seem to go wrong or look bad, I promise that I will not interrupt your process and take it back because of Doubt or I need Comfort. I will continue to press on and trust you. I want to increase in faith and in blessing. I want to glorify your name. Use me, empower me God! Take this situation, the burden and take control of it. It is in your hands!'

Security wrapped my heart and mind. I decided to leave it up to God. Things seemed to look up as I passed it into his hands. I may not have known what was going to happen, but I knew that I could trust God. I was going to be okay. As I had just heard the worst news of my life, I took the biggest step of faith in my journey with God and expected God to somehow do something amazing.

Response.

Finally, we have an answer. I was diagnosed with myelo-dysplastic syndrome. Relief was in place as the main feeling. I could move forward now after being stuck in the waiting room, filled with numerous blood donations and biopsies. The doctors and I moved forward, beginning to make plans to help me get onto the road of recovery. This was a massive shake up in my life, but I had a choice to either respond positively or negatively. I felt I should choose the former, as the latter does not help you do anything productively. Situations in our lives can hit us out of nowhere, or sometimes, like in my situation, we can see it coming from a mile away. One thing remains the same: there will always be situations we need to face. We cannot control that. We can control how we respond. It may take time to come to grips with what is happening, but ultimately, every situation requires a response from us—good or bad. A positive thought is that I knew God was walking with me, which I why

I handed the situation to him. This eased my burden and allowed me to feel safe in his hands.

Transference

March 2010. With the understanding that the Bone Marrow Transplant was the best step for me to recover, I was referred to a highly respected doctor, Dr Karin, at the Royal Children's Hospital. This was a huge blessing from God, knowing I was in great hands. Dr Karin took the opportunity to get to know me. She was very direct and had a presence that commanded the room. It might be age, experience, or respect. Either way, you knew when she was in the room. She had a low voice that conveyed strong meaning. Everything she spoke was out of knowledge of her field and understanding of the patient. Every time she listened, you knew she was present and attentive. Her thinking was very simple and practical. After getting to know her, I knew I was going to like having her as my doctor. Dr Karin organised another Bone Marrow biopsy to a more detailed analysis of how my condition was developing. They discovered that it was indeed getting worse and they gained more insight as to what my bone marrow was lacking: a chromosome was missing. Generally, we have twenty-three pairs of chromosomes to make forty-six. Chromosome number seven was missing a partner! This is common among those who have MDS, which can easily lead to Leukemia because the blood cells are not developing properly and immaturely.

Dr Karin began explaining the whole process of a Bone Marrow Transplant, sharing the measures they put in place to avoid/decreases risks. Dr Karin absolutely bombarded me with all the different types of risks there are involved in the transplant. There was a risk in the decrease of effectiveness of my organs, such as my heart. There was a chance of partial paralysis, a chance of needing a liver, kidney, or lung transplant if the bone marrow transplant affected those functions negatively. There was a chance that I could lose my eyesight, my hearing (even more so), my sense of smell, a sense of touch. A chance that the Bone Marrow Transplant may not even work, or I could have a relapse and end up back at square one. As she finished, she looked at me blankly, illustrating the seriousness of what was ahead and awaiting my permission. The different risks were flying through my mind as the immensity of the battle slowly unwound in front of me. There was a huge potential for fear to creep in as I imagined the battle ahead of me, but God laid a hand on my shoulder. '*Remember who I am and what I have promised you.'* These words counteracted all fear and eliminated all the conflicting feelings. I breathed out slowly and with peace. '*I understand, let us go ahead with it,'* I told my doctor. I spoke those words with no fear. God was on my side. Another faith step was made.

Registry.

My family were tested to see if they had a matching Bone Marrow set as mine, potentially being my donor. Strange thing was, it is very uncommon for family members to match; unlike an organ or kidneys. It is rare to have a matching donor in the family, while siblings have the highest chance with thirty percent. All my family members were told that they do not match my bone marrow. The fact that they were willing to be tested and potentially be my donor was a thought that did not go past my mind. The parameters for the search were made wider and my details were written into the Bone Marrow Registry, a database that compiles all the results of the people who have volunteered for a test to be a potential donor (shameless plug right there). I discovered the average time it takes for a donor to be found is twelve months. I did not want to play another waiting game so I turned to God and decided to make a deal with him. *In two months, by July, find me a donor or heal me.* He gave me a look that told me nothing, but communicated that he accepted the offer.

Testing.

To complete the preparations for the transplant, I was to be tested in all my vitals. This is done so that there is a reference point to go back to when I completed the transplant to see if I had recovered well or not. There were numerous appointments to book in. I had to get my eyes tested, my ears, my fitness, my heart, my lungs and my skin. At that point, I was still participating in my school studies for year eleven, just awaiting my number to be called up for hospital. I slowly spread the news that I was to have a Bone Marrow Transplant. The first people that found out were my extended family, close friends and church leaders. The most common initial reaction was shock and concern. I combated this by speaking with courage and assuring them that it was a good step, as I would be able to recover and be better than ever. It was heartening to see them believe my convictions and to know that I was in a friendship with God, who is greater than my circumstances.

Bet.

July 2010. I had another biopsy to see how my blood was progressing, or regressing. In another appointment with Dr Karin, she shared that all my blood counts and components were worse. The new blood cells that were flowing in my body were all immature blood cells and unable to maintain the functions of my body. I felt a slight loss of control. My body was a machine of its own that nothing I could do was going to help. It was a frustrating place to be in. Dr Karin had a rare slight grin. She announced that they had found a matching donor. With this supposedly great news, I turned to God: '*Oh no…now I have to follow through with this procedure.*' God smirked at me with an '*I-told-you-so*' look as he knew he had won the bet and poked fun of my foolishness in trying to make a deal with God. I swallowed my pride. Moral of the story: do not make deals with God, as he always wins.

Faint.

One Sunday morning, I was in church. I filmed someone who was speaking and then something began to feel a bit off. I was not sure what it was. I started to feel hungry. It seemed too sudden. I tuned into what my body was trying to tell me. A fuzzy sensation began swirling at the bottom of my stomach. It travelled further up, overwhelming my whole body. My head felt light and I knew something was going to happen. I moved away from the camera, turned around and before I know it, my head hit the ground with a thud; my body in a crumbled heap. I became unconscious. A thought came into my head a moment later: *James, what are you doing on the ground? Get up.* I opened my eyes gingerly and felt slightly embarrassed. People were surrounding me with panicked and concerned looks. One man had my head cradled onto the side so I could recover my rightful breathing rhythm. They held me there as my systems slowly regrouped and my thoughts regathered. I just fainted. It had never happened to me before. This is a new low that I have hit health wise. Would there be any more surprises like this? Did that mean I could go into public without a fear of fainting? It was a moment where I knew I was travelling in uncharted territory and my body was clearly getting worse. I was shaken up, as I did not know what was going to happen ahead. Dad took me to the hospital into the Emergency Ward. After being tested and checked upon, my blood tests revealed that my blood levels dropped to an alarming level, causing my body to take matters into its own hands and shut the system down temporarily. The instruction was to stay in hospital for a few days until my blood levels recuperated to a healthy standard.

Basketball.

Preparing myself to be placed in hospital for a long term and my derailing health, I played my last basketball for the season and for a while. It was quite upsetting because I was always active and had developed a love for the game, which I had started as a six year-old and never missed a season. Basketball was something that took my mind of what was going on. It was a passion and an outlet, yet it was being removed as I faced my biggest battle yet. I could not rely on basketball to help me get through the season of hardship. It was an enjoyable last game, however, as I was doing things out of the norm: playing tough defence, blocking three shots. Rare for a short bloke like me; and hitting my three-pointers. I surprised myself with this game due to the lack of energy I currently had. It was the understanding that I was not going to play for a while that gave me the extra fire and effort to leave it all on the court. It was a funny feeling as the game ended. I was joyous to have played with my team for a while and they gave me their well wishes. A door closed while I stepped into a new room; a room filled with the unknown.

Hickman.

In the week leading up to my seventeenth birthday in July, I was booked in for my Hickman Catheter to be inserted. It is a tube that goes inside your skin, beneath the armpits, trailing up inside your neck. It flows through into an artery that sits upon top of your heart. The purpose of the Hickman Catheter is to create a pathway for all the future transfusions that I would receive during this treatment: blood, platelets and poison (chemotherapy). This enables them to simply connect the transfusion needed to the line instead of continuously needing to jab needles into my veins each time. As I woke up after the Hickman line was inserted, an excruciating pain bulged on the side of my neck and my head felt heavy. It was as if I had been king hit. In this moment, the weight of the situation I was facing began to feel even more real. The reality of what was coming hit me: sickness, soreness and pain. To add to the growing list of appointments, I was instructed to go to the doctors each week to clean the wound from the Hickman line and change the dressing for a more sterile one to keep the area around my Hickman line disinfected. More visits to the doctors to add to my normal routine. Frustration was slowly building as I continued to wait for my number to be called.

During school, it was Wednesday, which meant I had a half day that day. I needed to go to three classes and then the hospital for my dressing change. I was feeling weak and lacking energy as I approached my classes. I knew my body was telling me something, but I convinced myself to push through, as there were only three classes. '*Suck it up James and it will be over soon.*' I built up the strength and attended. It did not bode well as I felt sicker and sicker. I was not even paying attention to class anymore. I focused on my breathing. It was heavy and I was trying to stabilize the breathing. *Breathe in, breathe out. Keep going.* My head began to spin and I realized it was a bad decision that I had made. I did not even have the strength to call out to the teacher that something was wrong. All my efforts were focused on trying to breathe and stay alive. The bell rang and the students happily packed up their books and moved out. A few students noticed that I am a bit out of it and grabbed the teacher's attention. As she was already aware of the circumstances I was facing, she rushed to my aid and took me to the sick bay area. My sister was called and she took me to the hospital. No words were spoken; I simply needed my energy to breathe. It was my priority. I arrived at the hospital and I could not get to the room fast enough. My body wanted to stop. My mind knew the destination was only a little bit further ahead. It was a conflict of feeling and need. I arrived into the ward and the doctors immediately took control of the situation.

I was so happy to allow my face to fall into a pillow and my body to rest and sink into the bed. I felt immensely sick and dehydrated. The doctors asked me questions to try and catch up to speed so they could take the necessary actions to rectify the situation. I was not being helpful because the last thing I want to do was talk. I was giving them yes and no answers to the best of my ability, which was not very good at that point. The doctors became concerned that my Hickman wound attracted a virus so they forced me to stay in observation for a few days. Not how I envisioned the rest of my week…It was discovered that my body became dehydrated because of a lack of sustenance and water. The price I paid was staying in a hospital bed, pumped with antibiotics, probed with testing, low level of entertainment, lack of Internet, and the all too well known, bad hospital food. As a day or two passed, I was bored out of my wits, restricted to playing games on my phone, watching movies on my laptop and sleep. I continually attempted to convince the medical staff that I was feeling okay. I asked to prove it by claiming that I could easily run a lap around the hospital. They continued to assert their authority that I needed to stay for observational reasons. I swallowed my stubbornness and yielded to their authority reluctantly.

Break.

It had been a week of staying at the hospital since my episode with dehydration. I knew that I was running out of time that I could spend with people before I went in for my treatment. This thought ran through my mind heavily and created frustration. God knew my desire to have a moment with my friends and people in my circle to give them some assurance that I was going to be okay, to give me assurance as I entered this mountain of a season; and to have a sense of pre-emptive goodbye, because I really did not know what the outcome would be. God, being the master-planner, enabled me an opportunity to leave the hospital for a few hours to see some people. My family drove up to attend my youth group for a little send-off. Our Youth Pastor, Ps Mike, shared a message based around 'letting it go'. It fitted perfectly to what I need to hear. It reminded me of everything that God was speaking into my life: to let go and let God take control. At the end, I was called to the stage. Ps Mike informed every person in the room of my situation; that I was going into hospital to get chemotherapy. He painted a very negative picture of the potential damage that chemotherapy can cause in your body. He created a negative tone and then, with great conviction, said, '*But this is not going to happen to James because God is with him.*' God wrapped me into his strong but gentle arms, covering me with strength and belief. Ps Mike and the rest of the youth prayed over my situation. Overwhelming me was this strange feeling that I was going to be okay. After all this, a friend came by and grabbed me by the arm with tears in her eyes. I reassured her that I was going to be back in no time and better than ever. I hugged her tightly. I still do not understand why I was so confident, but I understood that it was God's strength within me. This is the reassurance that I had been craving while in the hospital bed for the past week. I was aiming to leave because I needed to go back to hospital, but it took far longer because I was continually stopped in my tracks by people giving me their encouragement, prayers, assurance and hugs. It was an amazing feeling of being loved, assured and strengthened by others. God has truly created an amazing place of love, grace and relationships, all because we have encountered the amazing relationship we can have with God. Feeling full of the great love I received from others, and the massive assurance I received from God, we made our way back to the hospital. This time, I was refreshed.

Delay.

I was meant to be coming into hospital, but there was a delay due to logistical issues with the transportation of the Bone Marrow. It was frustrating because it meant that I had to keep doing school, even though I was becoming more fatigued and losing motivation, knowing that I was to be plucked out any moment; not finishing the semester. God reminded me of his perfect timing when it comes to plans. He reminded me that it worked in my favour because it increased my chances of jumping into the next year level above when I came back healthy because I had completed more of the semester. It allowed Mum to work a little more and take her personal leave from work at a better time with more hours. *If something is delayed, look closely as to why.* I smiled at God's assurance as I started this conversation grumbling and complaining... and finished it with a sense of purpose. *Just for you, I will keep pushing through this God. After all, you have never failed me yet!*

School.

As I knew that I was going to miss a large chunk of schooling, five months roughly, and no specific return date in mind, I needed to sort out my plan of how to keep up my schooling within reason. My family and I attended a meeting with a small group of staff from my high school. Ideas were shared and options thrown around. Deep down, I wanted to come back to school the next year after finishing my treatment and graduate with my friends, whom I had studied with all these years. I knew it was a far cry because the final year of high school is the most demanding mentally and emotionally. The option that was recommended was that I do my education via a correspondence company. To sum it up, it is a school that sends material and work, week by week, through mail and you complete the work required and send it back. I remember feeling quite reluctant to accept this option because something did not feel right. Mum felt quite concerned too because she wanted something more flexible; not strictly week by week. It made sense because anything could happen while I was going through the treatment. We left the meeting knowing the options presented and Mum began to ask God for direction; to know the most ideal method of education for my journey.

God pointed out that there was a Royal Children Hospital Education Institute. God clarified that they would be great to get more information from and a second opinion since they work with sick children of various sicknesses. We organised a meeting with an employee from the RCH Education Institute and shared our current options. He bluntly shared that we ought to not to do schooling via correspondence because it would be too much stress on myself as a patient/student. He rubbished the idea of it because it was complex to transfer mid-semester from school to Distance Education and vice versa. He threw a very good suggestion—*why don't you ask your current teachers if they can continue to teach you and send work out to you so you have more flexibility?* It made complete sense. This was a mini victory for me as that is what I wanted to do. It was fuss-free, no complications with transferences and the teachers knew me and my situation well. Only I needed to get the teachers on board if they were willing. We continued to follow the trail that God left us after we asked him for clarity in this situation. We presented the idea to the school and my teachers. They showed amazing support and generosity by agreeing to have my work sent out to me to the hospital. As a current student, it truly shifted my perspective. I often took them for granted because they constantly made me work, gave out homework, yelled at us when we only wanted to have a little fun. It was as if we painted them as the villains of our lives and we sought to antagonize them. Instead, teachers were assisting us in teaching us, trying to shape and strengthen each one of us to help build a better future and to help us establish ourselves in this world. These teachers became the supporters of my battle quickly by enabling me to see their desire for me to succeed in this fight. The school plans were agreed upon and sorted for the time being. August swung around and it was time for me to stop attending school and get started on transitioning to the hospital. The teachers held up their promise and sent me work to complete while I was assisted from a teacher from RCH Education Institute. All this was planned and done in hope that I could come back after the wilderness and complete year twelve. This became my goal in education and my motivation to push myself through—no matter what.

Night before.

My number was called up next to begin proceedings of the transplant. The night before was a calm before the storm. I had no idea what I was venturing into. The last year or two of my life had been building up to this treatment. In this treatment, anything can happen; so there was no point in worrying over It; otherwise it would have been too over-whelming. I spoke over my life and posted on social media as a form of assurance from God - *I may have been going through the toughest battle in my life, but it was merely an obstacle in God's plan.* These words brought comfort to me, as I knew in the long-term, everything would work out and I would be okay. It was a strange feeling; a sense of the unknown, but walking in with great confidence because I was entrusting everything with God. Perhaps this is what it means to have peace from God in the middle of every battle we face. There is a sense of knowing that I will be challenged in every aspect and I needed to prepare myself for this. Out of it, I would be strengthened in every aspect and be better than ever before. I prepared myself to sleep before the new season commenced the next day. My beautiful dog, Maggie, who is a small, territorial, Maltese cross poodle, jumped on my bed and slept the night there. It was as if she knew what was coming ahead. I laid there with her snuggled up by my chest. I knew that I ought to appreciate this night because I would not be able to play with my dogs for a few months minimum because my immunity was going to drop and I had to stay away from them to avoid attracting an illness. I held her close to me and the night was quiet, calm and peaceful. Maggie and I slept the night away, regardless of the immensity of the situation ahead. None of it mattered because I had God walking with me, my family supporting me; my church, youth and school cheering me on and praying for me. I slept with peace before the battle of chaos.

First Step.

To begin the proceedings, I had an appointment with Dr Karin. She gave me the run down on what I was going to receive for chemotherapy. She lays out some of the side effects of chemotherapy; which includes but is not limited to: lack of appetite, throwing up, hair loss, sore throat, weak muscles, ulcers and sores. I was a sponge, absorbing all the information she gave me, just nodding my head in return; praying for the best, and preparing for the worst. The aim of the first round of chemotherapy was to kill my current blood cells and decrease my immunity and enable the new bone marrow to be eased into my body system, creating its own blood cells. If it did not work out, my old cells could fight the 'foreign' bone marrow, causing the body to reject it. It is amazing how the body operates! Essentially, chemotherapy is putting poison in one's body to kill and destroy the blood cells and immune system.

I was taken into a shared ward, which consisted of two other patients. One was a young girl, six years old, seemingly in a small three year-old body due to a long battle with cancer and chemotherapy. It was heart-wrenching for me as I saw she had lost an eye due to a tumour. She had a few long strands of blonde hair left. It broke my heart to see a young girl have something we take for granted taken away at such a young age such as sight and still battle with issues. Every time medical staff came in, she unleashed a blood-curdling scream because she knew they were most likely coming with needles or something that caused her pain or discomfort. She associated them with negative experiences. She really inspired me; having to deal with all this at such a young age, starting life on the back foot. Most likely, having to prove nay-sayers wrong in the future with her sickness and lack of sight. I began praying for her, amid all this, that she would find God when she grew up, that she would have a better future than what most would assume; being moulded in strength from this tough situation. A thought hit me: if she could survive all this, then surely, myself, being older and stronger, could push through this.

First Dose.

As I received my first round of chemotherapy, the hospital stay was one week. I filled my time playing card games with other patients, did homework to keep my mind sharp and to keep track with year eleven studies and watched movies. There was a moment where I was watching a horror movie at night and a scene was taking place in a hospital. The curtains were pulled all around me for privacy and I was absolutely engulfed in this suspenseful scene, oblivious to what was around me. As I was watching it, I felt a massive hit to my bed and I flipped out. For a moment, I assumed that the monster was coming to get me and this is how it was to end for me. My bed copped another whack and I was scared out of my wits. It turned out that I had a flap attached to my bed and it was sticking out, causing the nurse to bump into it—not once, but twice!

The worse symptom that I had was no appetite, which was not too bad considering I could be throwing up, or be sore and weak. The medical staff marvelled at my initial progress, even though it was only the beginning. It felt great to know that my strength was showing, easing the pain of what was ahead, and it filled me with confidence; my conviction to remain sky-high. I smashed the first week of chemotherapy out of the park. Perhaps it was because my body was so sick for a long time leading up to it that it was adapting to being strong while sick; or it could have been God's hand over the situation, helping me to draw confidence from him. The medical staff completed their checks and give me the thumbs up to go home and rest before my next round of chemotherapy.

Negativity.

I stood in the kitchen and Dad walked up to me. He asked how I was going and I responded in a very confident fashion. I told him I was believing for a supernatural, speedy recovery, and the timeline which the medical staff had placed for my recovery was irrelevant. I shared with such conviction that God would overthrow the natural order in this battle so people could see that God's hand was over my life and in this battle. To my surprise, Dad completely rejected my ideals and stated that I should not expect God to do this. I needed to place certain measures and boundaries on this kind of thinking so I didn't get sick and disappointed. I stood in shock and soon, I woke up. I realized it was only a dream. I knew my Dad would not speak those words into my life as he is a faith-led man. This was Doubt trying to come into my thoughts, influencing negativity into my life by bringing a strong influence in my life in the form of my strong father into a dream and to cause me to reject my faith and the belief that I would be healed. Ironically, it only made me stronger, determined and driven to prove that I had the most powerful friend in the universe, God, who would help me overcome all this. I brimmed with confidence, resting in this assurance I placed over myself, despite the vivid dream.

Fever.

I woke up and the clock shone brightly into my dull eyes. It flashed three am. I was sweating profusely and alarms were going off in my head. My mouth was pained. I swivelled my tongue onto the wound, working out what the source and issue was. My mind was still waking up and playing catch up to the urgency of the situation. I realized that a massive ulcer had built overnight on the base side of my tongue. I alerted Dad and we quickly changed into suitable clothes; making the drive back to Royal Children's Hospital. Before I left the hospital earlier after finishing chemotherapy, the medical staff told me that my body would become feverish because my white blood cells were dropping and when that happens, I was to come back to the hospital immediately. That was it. The hospital provided us with a paper that had a specific set of instructions for the Emergency Ward Staff to follow considering I had very low immunity and my body was not equipped to fight hard and long. We arrived at the Emergency Ward and the staff were very quick and gracious in following the instructions and helping my body to settle and be brought under control. My medical staff came through the door and checked on me. They had commented so many times that I arrived at the perfect time. If it was any later, I would have been very sick. I thank God for ensuring everything ran smoothly and that I was safe in his hands. Then came the punch line: I was to stay in the hospital until my white blood cells climbed to a certain level, enabling me some form of protection against viruses. My mind groaned at the thought of this, but I understood the importance of it for my life.

Waiting Room.

The second stint in the hospital was definitely similar to being in the waiting room of life; the season between seasons, the place where your patience is tested, your discipline is built and you develop some sense of what is coming. It was a time where God was preparing me before the launch of what was coming. God prepared Mum with this encouragement, assurance and affirmation as she was preparing to be by my bedside for the next few months supporting me. As the days slowly passed, I lost a few kilograms. Mum, with a great sense of optimism, shared that I was indeed skinnier, but I looked great considering what was going on. My ulcer began to slowly heal as they were pumping me with antibiotics. However, the progress was too slow for me because I could barely eat or drink due to the pain on my tongue. Talk about missing the basic pleasures of life! I was finding ways to keep myself occupied, given I was in a small room with limited movement and visitors. There were movies, card games, social media, chatting to visitors, watching sports. I was still doing my schoolwork via mail to boost my chances of doing school that next year. I took up blogging too to help sharpen my mind, as well as share with my world my progress and how I was feeling. Best of all was sleep; it was the easiest way to kill time and not feel as much pain. It was like having a breather from a tough exercise—an off switch.

Hair.

One of the symptoms of chemotherapy began to kick in: my hair was slowly falling out. I grabbed my hair and it pulled out ever so smoothly. My mind had a little freak-out moment. *This is happening. I am losing my hair.* I look in the mirror and I saw that my whole fringe was gone because I had frantically pulled it out while I was panicking. As I lost a little confidence (in fact, a lot) because of my new look, God reminded me of Samson from the Bible. I felt a bit like Samson, losing my confidence as each strand continued to fall out; slowly losing the strength I had for this battle. Over the new few days, I was still losing my hair and was close to completely bald. I looked ten years older at least. It was a big reality check of the immensity of this battle. I knew I was not going to be able to coast through this like my first round of chemotherapy. The weight of this revelation sunk in deeper. God reminded me of Samson again. The strength I had did not come from me physically, or me being confident in how I was or how I looked (it certainly helped, but it is not the source). God was my source as he is the same yesterday, today, and tomorrow. God reminded me that he had promised me I would be okay. Knowing this, my confidence and strength ought to remain the same because my source never changed. A smile appeared on my face, bigger than ever. My confidence and strength was replenished by God. Besides, everyone gets a new look over time, right?

Inspiration.

Every day, as part of my routine, I had a walk through the hospital corridors with my portable monitor that kept track of my vital signs. The walk finished at the end of the corridor into a room where I could play card games with the hospital 'big brother', Micka, who spent time with kids to entertain them while they battled through their various challenges of illnesses. He worked for a company called Challenge, which was an amazing company that provided entertainment for kids, functions and charities to raise support, awareness, and morale among cancer battlers. During this walk, I crossed paths with a small boy who could not have been older than three. He looked up to me as I towered over him. He was bald too with no strands of hair sitting on his small head. He looked to me in shock and marvelled at my distinctive bald head too. He looked for a moment and moved his hand onto his head, showing his astonishment that we had something in common. In his eyes, he felt warmth as if he was looking at his inspiration; someone who was bigger, stronger, yet going through the same thing he is. However, for me, he was my inspiration! Someone who was smaller, younger, yet powering through something that I was going through as well. It was a touching moment. I grabbed a hold of his hand and nodded at him with a big smile on my face. I did so in confidence that we both would be okay and stronger than ever. That moment served as a reminder of the bigger picture of what I was going through; a reminder that I would beat cancer and as a result, inspire others through this story. That moment galvanised me with newfound clarity and strength, knowing that I could impact others through this situation, to give people encouragement that they can beat their circumstances. My family, friends and acquaintances continually shared that they were encouraged and inspired by my fight and my attitude towards this situation. All these things were adding fuel to my fire to push past this battle and succeed.

New Life.

September 2010. A blessing arrived in the middle of my battle for my family. My aunty had delivered her first child, Lola. My mother was ecstatic to be an aunty on her side of the family. It was so handy to have something to take our mind off what was happening in my situation and have something to defuse the stress or burden momentarily. To be able to feel joy, to celebrate new life in this world, a new addition to the family, to reflect on the good things in the world that we can often fail to stop and ponder. Going through what I was battling through; experiencing it first hand, or secondarily, it was so easy to be caught up in the gloom of it all. So easy to be burdened by the 'what ifs', the questions it brought, the uncertainty it held. For me, life brings what life brings, I could only do the best I could do with it. The best for me was to follow God who had my back, to look at the blessings he had brought me, to build the strength and faith I needed to overcome this, and to take joy in the moments I could. A simple smile in this battle had become so powerful. I could not wait to meet my new cousin one day soon.

Detained.

Since I came back to Hospital due to my fever, the only thing detaining me was the wait for my white blood cells, called Neutrophils, to increase to give me some form of immunity protection while I was at home. This wait was far longer than we all expected. My neutrophil count was simply not growing. It was testing my patience and my faith in the process. The time in hospital was starting to gnaw at me as I spent most of my time playing games, watching television and chatting to the people who were looking after me. Every day, I wait eagerly for my blood test and their results. Every day, the nurse would share that they had not increased. The waiting room season was bringing its challenges.

Faith and Blessing

While waiting in hospital, Mum began to share about how God was providing specific needs. A short time before my hospital stay, mum was scratching her head with what to do for her many accumulated months of work leave. Now, she could take her leave to look after me, while being paid by work, easing any financial stress on the family. Sure, she would have loved better circumstances, but life threw this situation at us and she was given the favour of providence. Mum shared that she was also blessed with an extra four weeks carer's leave from work, totalling to six months paid leave. God's hand was truly upon this situation. It bolstered my confidence in my decision to trust that God had everything under control. I decided to take my faith one step further. I wanted to test my faith and thinking when it came to believing for the unlikely. Since my health diagnosis, I had been told of the procedure, what it involves, and the risks associated to it. The medical staff shared that the process was two weeks of chemotherapy over a four-week period, the transplant and six months, minimum, to a year of recovery. These were the facts presented in front of me. I ask God how he can come through for me in a spiritual aspect and turn the situation on its head a little. God gave me his word that I would be healed in six months, completely. The hair on my neck stood up a little at this thought. *Six months? That's in February? You sure?* I questioned God a little bit to get more out of him. *Trust me, write everything down and believe in it.* I did not know how this was going to happen, but this is where the stretch in faith kicked in. I wrote it down and begin believing that I would be recovered within six months, back at school next year doing year twelve, and graduating with all the people I have done the past five years with. It all looked very unlikely, but this was God's opportunity to shine his light over my situation and bring something great into fruition. I had a meeting with my doctor and shared my newfound goal. She shut it down immediately. *James, there is absolutely no chance of you going back to school in February with this process. You ought to put all your focus on your health. This is of utmost importance.* I completely understood where she was coming from. However, this gave me more motivation to take care of myself, see this promise from God come to fruition, and prove people wrong. I laid down these plans for my timeline and education and continued to allow God to do what he needed to do and continually asked God to let me know what I needed to do.

Neutrophils Rising.

I was now three weeks into my stay at the hospital since I got the fever after my first round of chemotherapy. I was losing confidence and patience, as there were no signs of growth in Neutrophils. My mother and I decided to do something for the fun of it. We heard that there was a strong case of God's genius at work when it came to natural foods and body parts. There was a theory that certain fruits and vegetables can assist certain functions of specific body parts in which it closely resembles. For example, a walnut looks like a brain and it can aid in warding off dementia, can help rid of plagues associated with Alzheimer's. A tomato resembles a heart and claims to be as pure heart/blood food. A sliced carrot looks like an eye and can increase blood flow to eyes, decreasing chances of cataracts. Sussing this thought out, my mother bought grapes and I began to eat them all day because grapes can resemble blood cells and apparently, they have nutrients that can assist blood cells. I ate grapes over the next couple of days. The nurse came in, bustling with an ounce of good news each day. The Neutrophils count were slowly increasing and multiplying. After the third day, my Neutrophils count finally grew from 0.3 to 0.5, which was the target. The nurse took me off antibiotics and gave me permission to go home and enjoy my last week before I came back for more chemotherapy. Whether the increase of the count came from the grapes or more vigorous prayers to God, we will never know. All I knew was that I was continuing to trust that God had me in his hand for I had entrusted the situation to him.

Risk.

Coming home, there was a huge risk, as I currently had an extremely low blood count and immunity. I was bald and I had nothing to protect myself from viruses or flues that would hamper my recovery or delay my transplant. Extra care was required from myself, my family and others. After a four week stay at the hospital, I had a bucket list of things to do before I went back, but the majority of them never happened because of roadblocks. It was as if God was protecting me from any issues. The first item was that I planned to say good-bye to some school friends on the last day of the term, but there arose a last-minute request for a blood top up which made me stay at the hospital for an extra three hours, blocking me from catching my friends at school. Another item was that I wanted to say farewell to my friends from youth, but the plan also fell through due to a miscommunication. Another item was that I wanted to meet my new cousin, but on that day, she ended up with conjunctivitis, which was a big risk for me. Lastly, I wanted to have a movie night with a big group of people, but there were only two that could make it because of colds, flues and family visiting. Those two were my best mates and I ended up having a fantastic, quiet night with those two. After all these subsequent events happened over the week and the challenges that came with trying to tick off my bucket list, I realise that if I looked at what I wanted and it did not come to fruition, I would wonder where God was. If I looked at the big situations and worked out where God was, I may not have found him because God is a God who works in the small and finer details. As I considered all the 'coincidences', I could say that God was working to keep me safe and to ensure I was protected. This gave me the assurance that God was with me and the courage to continue to trust in him every step of the way. Despite all the risk involved, the trust in God was paying off and I was growing very close to God as he beckoned me on forward.

Preparation.

October, 2010. I was making my final preparations for my stay in the isolation room, which is called the 'Fish Bowl', for my last round of chemotherapy, and eventually, the bone marrow transplant. I had shaved off the remaining hairs off my head and adopted the bald look confidently. I happily received compliments and knew I was in good stead for the future should I lose my hair under better circumstances of age. I was blessed with the honour of winning the 'Monash Inspirational Award', which is an award given to a person battling cancer whom is showing great courage and determination. It was a reminder of the greater picture of why I was going through this situation, as God brought back my first words from him: *I will have a life-inspiring story that would change people's lives.* The great part was that the award came with a financial grant. The majority of the finances went to paying for a new close buddy of mine for my stay to keep me occupied in isolation: a Playstation! Along with the Playstation, I had a TV, movies and a laptop to keep me sane in hospital.

Visitors.

I was nearly set for my stay in isolation. The medical staff revealed that I was only allowed to have four people to become regular visitors for my stay in isolation to limit any setbacks. Naturally, I choose my parents and my sister, as they would be journeying the closest to me. My mother had finished work and was entering a new chapter of being my carer in this critical season. It was so good to be reminded of God's provision due to the fact that she was still receiving pay from work. I knew that mum would be challenged and moulded by God to increase in wisdom and stature as she continued to trust in God also. I had one more spot left. There was a debate to who should take up the valuable final spot until someone jumped at the opportunity when he heard It was available. Steve, who was my youth co-ordinator, had grown close to me the last few months as he supported me over the journey thus far. Steve always ensured that he had the latest updates with my progress. He continually prayed for me and kept everyone at youth and church updated. Steve, with great eagerness, asked if he could take the last spot as a member outside of my family. I knew Steve was God-sent so I accepted without any hesitation. From that moment, Steve became a pivotal part of the battle. He became the big brother that I could draw wisdom, joy and fun from. The irony was that despite not going through cancer himself, Steve had endured some hospital process that I was going through and was able to relate to my level, giving me some encouragement, affirmation and a peace of mind.

Looking back, this was an amazing sacrifice for Steve, considering he was working two jobs at the time, engaged to his fiancé, along with co-ordinating a youth program and fixing up the new home he was moving into once married. He made this situation work because he had every motivation to show his love and support in my battle. This thought alone was humbling and caused me to be so grateful and appreciative of his sacrifice.

Round Two.

Heading into my second round of chemotherapy, I was feeling very confident that I could smash through this round just as I did my last one with minimal symptoms. What I did not realise was that my body was far more weakened after the underlying impact of less blood cells, less immunity and overall, less strength to fight. As I went through the first couple of doses, I was absolutely hammered by all the side effects of chemotherapy. I felt ill everywhere in my body, from my head, to my throat, to my stomach. I had absolutely no appetite and I couldn't even force myself to eat because I felt even more sick at the thought of eating. I ached in every single muscle I had in my body, feeling weak and not wanting to move. My mouth hurt due to many ulcers developing and making camp there. It stopped me from talking because my throat burned as I made an effort to speak. I was thirsty, but water did not taste good due to the irritations in my mouth and throat. The best medicine for drinking was cold cordial. I took sips of it and made minimal effort to swallow to ensure ease of pain as it went down my throat. I was hooked up to a specific dose of morphine to assist the pain, but couldn't have too much, or else otherwise I would overdose. It felt like the morphine did absolutely nothing as my body ached and groaned away while they fed me more chemotherapy through the tubes into my body. I just wanted relief. Sleep became my greatest escape. Every time I slept, my mind did not think about the pain, the agony, or the situation I was in. It was like I was running off to another world temporarily, only to wake up to the fact that I was still in reality facing my battles. I began to sleep as much as I could because it was the only time I felt okay and it helped pass the time effortlessly. I began sleeping around twenty to twenty-two hours a day! Mum was by my side, tending to my needs every small waking moment I had. She was killing time by watching television series, journaling and having coffee with some visitors when they dropped by.

Prayers.

Mum routinely informed me of people who were praying for me. The circle of people praying was growing bigger and bigger. I was amazed at the love and care from people who were regularly keeping me in their prayers. She informed me that Nana and Granddad had a large group of people from the Salvation Army gathering and praying for a person they did not know. My church was praying, my family was praying; people who did not believe in God are praying, which did not make sense to me. Maybe it helped, for they did not know who they were praying to, but prayers were still lifted for my sake. I was overwhelmed by this thought. Mum illustrated the impact perfectly: *it was like a prayer blanket was covering you, keeping you warm and safe.* I rested in this thought with great confidence. God smiled alongside my bed in acknowledgement that he was hearing those prayers and that I was going to be okay.

Dreams.

Since sleep was my only escape, and I was sleeping a lot, it seemed that I kept having reoccurring dreams. The same two dreams happened over, over, and over again. Imagine watching a short movie every single time that you become afraid to turn on the television again because you do not want to see the same movie on. There was a sense of symbolism however, in those two dreams. I remember every single detail as it is etched in my mind.

In the first dream, *it was pitch black outside, bucketing with rain. Horrendous conditions. There was a long line of broken down trucks, lining up before a mechanic's garage on a moving strip. I could hear the clanking and moaning of these large machineries. There was a moving walkway that each truck was placed on. These trucks were being moved towards the garage slowly and stopped as each machine entered the garage, one by one. My focus was on a beautiful red truck that had the front ripped upside down and was disconnected from the back storage. Once the trucks spent a few moments in the garage, which you couldn't see inside because of these big, tinted black windows, they were slowly shipped outwards and they were fixed. These machines went out the other side, as beautiful as ever. The red truck finally entered the garage, waiting to be restored in all its glory again.* This dream felt strange, but through this, God assured me that he is in the process of fixing me up, restoring me to my original self; that I would be okay. I kept waking up frustrated because it was the same dream every time I closed my eyes. It was the same repetition, like a thirty second clip over and over. But I did grab an understanding of the affirmation it brought, with the symbolism of creation and renovation. This dream assured me that everything was going to be okay, as I had the master mechanic in God working on me. I would be okay.

Every other time I closed my eyes, I found myself going dizzy from another repetitive dream, one that was far, wild and engaging. *I was in this heavenly meadow—mountains, big and wide. Hills short and high. Everything was covered in greenery. I took a big breath and freshness entered my senses. As I looked around, hills were all spread out and no end was in sight. It was limitless. Accompanying me was beautiful weather, sun shining bright; not too hold or cold, perfect. I had never been enchanted by nature as much as I was now. There was serenity and peace residing in the atmosphere and within my heart. I walked a few steps and started jogging as I garnered momentum. I leaped with all my might and flew higher than I had ever been before. I landed on a higher mountain with such grace, coming to a rolling stop. I leaped off again and soared down like an eagle to the lower hills, to another rolling stop. The movements seemed effortless. Each landing had amazing finesse; rolling over like I was the greatest gymnast. There was such fluidity in my motions. It was exhilarating. I continued jumping, leaping, rolling, soaring with such freedom and vigour. Consciously, every time I landed, I kept telling myself to calm down, relax, stop jumping around as I felt myself becoming dizzier in my natural sleep. But something within me did not want to stop. This was an amazing place and this was an incredible sensation: to fly, soar and jump with no limitations and with such elegance. Joy within me bubbled to the surface. I had a huge smile on my face and shouted roars of delight every time I flew.* I woke up feeling like I had done a workout each time this dream popped up. I could sense my heart rate attempting to slow down after a thrilling dream experience. I began to wonder why my dreams were so repetitive, and why these two specific dreams? God turned to me and brought me fresh insight. This dream was a window to the waiting room where my spirit resides as my body was going through this natural procedure. My spirit had time and room to refresh and move freely. God had given this heavenly meadow in my dream to allow my spirit to be re-energized. My mind was blown away at this concept, but I did not doubt the idea. It did bring a sense of energy to myself and I will never visually forget this. I closed my eyes and instantly remembered the place with ease. It was a snapshot of perfection.

A new dream finally popped up on the reel as I continued to sleep away time. *I was sitting on the bench of a basketball game. I was fully decked out in my basketball uniform, waiting with such eagerness to jump on. I was bouncing with energy, bustling with spirit. I craved to jump onto the court and run around. I finally got my number called up and I ran with such passion. My muscles twitched as I was in the game, diving, running, evading, shooting and defending.* I woke up calm, feeling like my body had been worked and my desire to play had been quenched. The signals in my body were alert and alive as I dreamt I was playing. My body and mind was really providing avenues for me to keep my senses sharp and my desires intact as I lay down in my bed; sick, sore and lazy. Sleep and dreaming continued to sucker-punch reality each time. I used every motivation to continue sleeping as much as I could, as I found the days were going slightly faster.

Sister.

My sister was currently doing her most important year of high school education, her final year. There were many exams, assignments and work for her to do. On top of this, her brother was going through cancer. We ensured that we kept her focused on this year of school, without being too distracted with what I was going through, despite it being an immense situation. This often led to her feeling a little out of the loop when it came to involvement with me. She was finally coming today for the first time since I had returned for chemotherapy, but it was not a good time. I had developed such bad ulcers, all clustered in my throat and on the back of my mouth. I couldn't talk or swallow without feeling pain. I spent those days not talking, unless necessary. She came into the room and I caught a little look of anguish on her face, even though she tried to hide it. *I could not talk.* I used all my tolerance to tell her this sentence to give her a heads up. She began to make conversation and all I could do was nod my head and listen. She was pretty much talking to a brick wall. It was an interesting situation because she had seen me grown up fit, sporty, active and enthusiastic; now I was weak, tired, sore, mute. As the session wrapped up, I was so proud to have my sister. It was a commendable effort to push through this final year of schooling while supporting me through this battle. Such character. She inspired me to continue to push through myself, no matter what I faced.

Painful Visit.

As I was still not willing to talk because of the pain, Steve came in for his routine visit and this felt like a gruelling session because I could not converse or engage with him. Steve did a fantastic job to put on a smile and talk about whatever he could think of; despite the limited replies. I felt frustrated because I was passionate about engaging with others, but I couldn't do so in this shape. I began to feel like a burden; that these people are here to babysit me, talk to me about pointless things. But I also felt blessed. Steve was actively putting in effort to ensure that I was as comfortable as I could be in this situation. He was fuelling up my spirits through his wisdom, laughs and presence. After an hour passed, Steve prayed for me and asked if I need anything. I told him I was fine and he departed till next time.

Mess.

My body was not functioning well anymore due to the lack of white cells and nutrients that help any daily body activity. I had 'the runs' downstairs and absolutely no bowel control. It was as if my dignity was slowly being stripped away. I asked my mum to buy a bulk pack of underwear because I kept having small accidents and I needed to ensure I was keeping myself clean. My bathroom was only a couple of metres away from me, but I only had under a minute to react to get my bottom onto a toilet bowl to ensure a clean passageway. The process of getting there often resulted in messy consequences because either my mind was too slow to react, or my body did not have enough control to hold the movements, even for just a second. I ended up changing my underwear up to three times a day. To make matters more difficult, as I was hooked up to a vital signs monitor, with cables going into my body for fluids, chemotherapy and so on, there were so many different plugs attached to the machines, meaning I must pull them all out to enable me freedom to move and take my attachments with me to the bathroom… every single time I needed to go.

One night, I was sleeping and I felt the subtle alarm bells ringing in my head. I woke up and it was two in the morning. My body was frantically alerting me that I needed to go find a toilet. My mind was still groggy and trying to correspond. I rolled out of bed and proceed to pull out all of the cables. To add to the frustration, the cables did not budge. I was pulling, my muscles tensing up; then my body warned me, *Too late! I am going now!* Acting on my instincts, I looked around quickly and I saw a bin a few steps ahead. I rushed towards it, yank my pants down and excrements exploded out. As I finished, I looked around and gazed in horror. Only a small amount made it into the bin, but the rest was scattered across the wall, outside the bin, and on the floor. I sighed in disgust and frustration. All I cared about that moment was that I got it out of my system. After cleaning myself up, I sat on the bed. I rested my head on my palm, wondering how long this was going to go for, and how low this experience kept getting. I swallowed my embarrassment and buzzed the nurse in. She walked in and I explained the situation to her. She responded understandingly and proceeded to collect the appropriate tools to clean it up. I felt slightly better after receiving the support from the nurses and no shame was given. It was all part of the process.

Since the 'explosive' accident, I decided that it was getting too risky for me to rely on making it into the bathroom in time with the limited strength I had, with all the hooks and cables accompanying me. The medical staff agreed and they provided a toilet bedpan to sit on the chair just a few steps away from me. I felt much safer in going about my business, and less worried about the situation from repeating itself.

Catheter

A side effect of the type of chemotherapy dose I was receiving was potential poison in my kidneys, unless I peed it out of my system quick enough. To ensure that my kidneys were in good shape, the nurses had to assess my pee. They shared that I needed to have a catheter (a tube) inserted into my 'willy'. I shuddered at the thought of this, but health simply had to come first. I was feeling nervous about this appointment; I was anticipating all the different scenarios. *What if it hurts? What if I pee while they put it in?* The nurse came in all smiles, despite the awkwardness surrounding my thoughts. The nurse assured me and explained the situation. *It will only feel uncomfortable for a short moment*, she told me. Before I knew it, she guided the catheter into the opening of my appendage and allowed it to reach into my bladder. My whole body held its breath during this untraveled experience. After a few moments of grimacing, it was completed. I let out a big sigh of relief. The tube was attached to a bag, referencing how much it had been filled. The most frustrating incidents were when I needed to go to the toilet and the cable wasn't big enough to carry all excessive urine at such a swift speed, so it would often burst around and past the cable and explode out, causing it to be painful. Since I had a bag at the other end too, each time I went, I had to manoeuvre the tube around my underwear before I got on with my 'business'. The catheter was in my system for two days while I received this specific type of chemotherapy. I was happy to see the end of it, as it became one less problem for me to have to worry about. I felt sick and sore; I was enduring the runs while receiving chemotherapy. I sensed my body slowly being pushed to the brink of death, with all the nutrients inside wallowing in poison. My dignity was being stripped away each day, safe to say that I wanted it to stop, be over, and go home. I wanted to have it over and done with.

Assassin

It was near the end of my round of chemotherapy. The nurse came in with a new batch of chemotherapy. It seemed different to the others: black in colour and looking to blow out of its seams. *This is your last one James! She told me.* The nurse gave me the good news, then proceeded with the bad. *This was the biggest, baddest of all chemotherapy. It was the brew that would literally murder the body cells and finish the job for us. It is the deadly assassin that will never fail.* My body was in horrible shape from all the previous treatment of chemotherapy. I thought I had this in the bag after my first round, but now my confidence was in the ditches. I was throwing up, sick in every way, shape, and form. They hooked me up to the final mix of chemotherapy and I endured it over the next two days. Sleep was my only escape, but I was struggling to gain peaceful rest. I felt worse than a marathon runner who hits the brick wall half way through his race. I had never been so exhausted, nor in agony, as I have at this point. I remembered the moment a month before this battle what I wrote on social media—*I may be facing my toughest battle in life, but it is merely an obstacle in God's plan.* These words smacked me in the face like a cake. I was eating my words after thinking it was going to be easy! All my focus was put into simply getting through this two days of torment.

Carried.

It was the third morning since I had been hooked up to the horrid last chemotherapy dose. I woke up with an even worse throat and a disgusting taste filled my mouth. An ache pounded against my head as I came to my senses. I looked down to an itch on my tummy and noticed a massive rash had formed. I refused to continue my waking moments and decided to close my eyes and fell asleep again to help the ignorance of what was occurring. A new dream occurred on the REM playlist. *There was a dirt track and I was laying down, a broken, crippled figure. I uttered a cry for help to God. It began to feel like an end. I was done. An arm reached under my back. I flinched for a moment. The other arm moved under my leg, cradling me. Effortlessly, the figure picked me up. I noticed it was Jesus himself. I couldn't quite get a clear picture of him as my eyes were fatigued and not adjusting to the dim morning. Intuitively, I knew it was Jesus. Jesus walked up the trail, gaining ascendency with each step. Within moments, we reached the top of the mountain. Jesus lay me to the ground and propped my body up so that I could see the view. It was bewildering. I allowed this moment to saturate my every being. Jesus began to explain that my body had this amazing ability to adapt to the circumstances it was struggling with. Jesus cited the examples of myself when I was first ill with the bone marrow, resulting in low stamina; yet my body continued to work out a way for me to keep participating in basketball and other rigorous activities. Jesus shared a situation from a long time ago when I was twelve; how my foot had developed a cluster of warts underneath the big toe and it was too painful to walk. Yet, my body found a way to walk with minimal pain possible. As Jesus shared these examples, he comforted me with the promise that mine and everyone else's prayers of a speedy recovery would be answered. Just trust in the body's uncanny ability to adjust. Then Jesus hit me with an even better promise; six words I will never forget.*

"This is your last one ever"

I woke up. It took me a while to figure what he was referring to. My brain was mush at this point. I think he was going to leave me in my suspension, then I realised what it was in reference to—chemotherapy! This was my last day of chemotherapy, ever! Joy overcame me in my state of illness. My heart felt warm to know such a great friend in God, who cared for me immensely. I held onto these words as if they were bound to my heart forever as a promise from God. I gained insight to the big picture that brought encouragement. God was going to touch the hearts of others because of the battle I was facing. I did not need to feel anything because God had my back. I was going to be okay; more than okay. I was going to conquer this. Warmth serenaded my body as I rested in this state of mind.

Marrow.

Chemotherapy was finished. A refreshing fragrance filled the room. Today was a day off before the new bone marrow attempts to make its home in my system. There were some unusual circumstances in which my bone marrow had come to be in my hospital room. My donor was a French woman. *Bonjour!* It was by chance that a doctor from my medical staff was having a short holiday in France and she decided to pick up the bone marrow matter with her, flying home from France with my new bone marrow matter. This meant that it would be even fresher considering it did not have to go through all the processes of handling, but would come straight to the hospital room I was in. Prayers were lifted by everyone I knew for a safe flight and journey for the bone marrow transplant. As the bone marrow arrived, the staff conducted the final testings to ensure the bone marrow indeed matched my own numbers. In order for the foreign bone marrow to be accepted by the host's body, the numbers needed to match in three different faucets minimum out of six. The bone marrow originally matched mine in four areas. As they conducted the final testings, the numbers actually matched in five out of six! Talk about favour! It was near perfect and freshly arrived, straight from the source. God was definitely working his magic to provide the best bone marrow for me. It was impossible not to feel safe in God's arms and provision.

Mishap.

In the final day before my bone marrow transplant, I noticed that the staff had been continuously adding more tubes to my Hickman Line. (the catheter that was under my armpit as a gateway for the blood, platelets, and essential nutrients I needed for my body) The staff were adding more tubes because they were giving me more nutrients. It got to the point that whenever I travelled outside of my bed, I had to hold the weight of the tubes, as they were getting heavy. I assumed it was normal and part of the process. That night, I woke up from a lovely sleep and went to the restroom. As I entered the door, something felt odd. My mind was still waking up as I try to work out what felt off. I couldn't put my finger on it. I notice red spots plopping onto the floor. My brain finally caught up with the situation and I realized that my Hickman Line had fallen out from my armpit, despite the tape, because of the weight. Blood began gushing out like crazy and panic overwhelmed me. I did the one thing I knew I ought to do: I quickly covered the wound and placed pressure on it. I buzzed in the nurse to alert them. They were surprisingly quick and reacted fantastically to quite a mishap. I sat on my bed while they covered the wound, cleaned the mess, and started discussing a plan on how to transplant the bone marrow into my system, considering the main gateway to my body was now gone. My thoughts betrayed me as I asked questions to God. *Why now? So close to the transplant, why now?* I was presented with two choices. To panic and doubt God's work, or to trust in God and believe everything would work out. I only had five hours before the scheduled infusion of the bone marrow. I remember the promise I made to God when I gave him the situation. *I promise that I will not interrupt your process and take it back because of Doubt.* I chose the latter and trusted in God. Calmness surrounded me, despite what occurred abruptly, something that could have thrown a lot into chaos. The nurse came up with a plan and inserted the lines into my hand and arm manually for the bone marrow transplant. They booked me into surgery after the scheduled bone marrow transplant to get a new catheter inserted under my other armpit. The only downside was that the surgery meant I had to fast food and drink for the whole day on the day of my bone marrow transplant in preparation for anaesthetic surgery. Mum figured out a way to find a blessing in disguise and exclaimed *Praise God for a new line to allow the bone marrow to be as fresh as possible while traveling to your body!* There is a silver lining in everything. I had a bone marrow fresh off a plane, increasing in compatibility to my body and now a fresh line to go with it. I was ready for the transplant.

Zero.

It was day zero. The day of the transplant, which we had been counting down to. All the appointments, medical check-ups and chemotherapy had been building up to this day. There was a little celebration as my family, my medical staff and myself knew that the way from here was upwards. The nurse checked all my vitals and my systems to ensure everything was all good to go, especially after the mishap the night before. We got the A-Okay and the nurse hooked me up to my new bone marrow and the bone marrow started making its way into my body. On its journey to discover my bone marrow, it made its home there and started to multiply, eventually developing the healthy blood system my body needed to function well. The waiting game continued as it would take its time.

Complication.

I noticed a couple of strange sensations happening. At noon, my tongue swelled out for a moment. I could not draw it back into my mouth. Within a minute, it was back to normal. I notified the doctor, but they shrugged it off since there were no visible signs or changes. I was trying to watch a football game as I passed the time, but frustratingly, my eyes were blinking, involuntarily, at a rapid rate. As they blinked, my eyes were getting tired, but I couldn't sleep because they continued to blink while I was attempting to sleep. Talk about a polarizing effect! I grew wearier as the day passed by. The football game was of no interest to me anymore as my mind was occupied with how fatigued I was feeling, yet frustrated because I couldn't sleep. My body was still in a weakened state from the battering it copped throughout chemotherapy. I was a depressed figure because I couldn't enter my escape with sleep. At five o'clock, I felt that something was happening to my body, but I did not want to make a big deal. I just wanted sleep. Rest. I said my goodbyes to Mum as she left for her routine time. She asked if I needed anything. I shook my head and quickly brushed her off. As she left, I buzzed my nurse in. I asked if I could have some sleeping pills because all I wanted to do was sleep. I was surprised as she gives them to me without hesitation. It must have been within my parameters of my circumstances that they were aware of. In my hand, I held two sleeping pills that would bring me the most beautiful and anticipated sleep in all its awaited glory. I moved my hand to my mouth and attempted to swallow the pills. In an instant, something crazy happened. My throat immediately clogged up and my tongue swelled up again, making it impossible for me to swallow the pills. I knew something was happening, but I was frustrated because I simply wanted to sleep. If I could have had those pills and slept, I would be happy, even if it meant I did not wake up again. I was tired; I did not want to fight anymore. Sleep evaded me in this moment. I threw the sleeping pills onto the ground. I gathered my breath as I anticipated everything was about to become crazy. I buzzed the nurse in and once she saw the state I was in, she called in the whole medical team. It was officially an emergency that required all hands on deck.

I couldn't talk properly considering I had a beast of a tongue propped out of my mouth. I mumbled my way through questions. I couldn't hear anything because I did not have my hearing aids in. Talk about a difficult patient. I gathered that the nurse was asking if I request anyone's presence. I managed to ask for Dad and they called him. As he was on his way, I saw the staff flicking through thick medical books for any insight to what was occurring. They stabbed me with injection after injection on prayers, hoping that each was an answer to counteract what was occurring in my body. Nothing was subduing the effects. They gave me an oxygen mask to assist me in breathing with the clogged throat. It was so uncomfortable with my swollen tongue, so I kept trying to brush it off, but the nurses kept on readjusting it to ensure I was getting my oxygen. My eyes were tearing up because of the continuous rapid blinking. It was harder for me to see clearly. Dad made it in record time and the medical staff proceeded to take me to the Intensive Care Unit (ICU) because something needed to be done and done quickly. It was a tricky situation as I was in isolation so they needed to transfer me with care and minimal traffic as possible. I was passive, being a human dummy as they worked out what the issue was. The answer came: it was discovered that I was having an anaphylactic attack in response to the last chemotherapy substance that was dosed into my body. It is a rare occurrence to react this way, and to have a delay in the reaction; hence the length of time it took to figure out the issue. Anaphylactic attacks usually occur from insect bites, bee stings, food allergies, or in my case, medication.

ICU

As I entered ICU, the team pumped me with fluids to flush out all the substances that were injected into me earlier. My heart rate was rapid; my blood pressure was high. My tongue was swollen. I was dehydrated as I couldn't swallow water. My throat kept pushing it back up. I had teary eyes and couldn't see properly due to the involuntary blinking that was becoming faster. Lastly, I was delirious. I kept seeing six to eight people in the room, tending to me. Due to the fluids being pumped into me at a fast rate, I needed to pee every ten minutes. Every ten minutes, I would shout to everyone to leave because I needed to go to the toilet. To me, they took forever to get out. I had a jug in my hand and it was a challenge to get myself sorted out to pee in the jug. Once I finished, they all came back in and resumed their work. It turned out that there was only one medical staff and my dad in the room! Effects of delirium right there…The fluids continued to pump through my tubes; the uncomfortable oxygen mask remained over my mouth. Things continued to go from bad to worse. I couldn't drink water, thus becoming more dehydrated. The pupils of my eyes began to shift towards the left side.

I tried swinging them back to their natural state in the middle, but they flung back each time. Fear began to overwhelm me. *What if I am like this for the rest of my life? What if I become a healthy minded person, trapped in a crippled body, not able to communicate or move as I did before?* It was real fear that began to attack my mind in this critical circumstance. There was a moment of choice. Do I submit to these fears, or stand firm on God's promise? My dad was doing everything he could to assist; providing me the jug for pee, keeping me hydrated, and knew, despite my deafness, that I could hear a little if he spoke directly into my ear. I cried out to Dad and mumbled the words, *Am I going to be like this for the rest of my life?* He replied calmly with a no. In an instant, I was comforted. Never had one simple word been so powerful in a moment that eradicated all my fears instantly. My mind readjusted its focus and I meditated on God's promise. *He's got my back. I can get through this, and overcome it.* Dad found a face washer. He soaked it with warm water and placed it over my eyes. *Sleep, D*ad encouraged me. *I was reminded of the story of Jesus healing a blind man in the Bible (John 9:17). Jesus stoops down, picks up a pile of dirt. Spits in it, creating mud. Jesus places it over the man's eyes. The man's eyes begin the process of being healed completely.* There was fantastic parallels symbolism between these two situations. I felt God's hand over me throughout this current battle, working through me and strengthening me in every moment I needed it. As I attempted to sleep,

I struggled as my eyes continued to blink. I opened my eyes again. *I can't sleep. My eyes are still blinking.* I expressed my frustration to Dad. *Try again.* Dad continued to affirm me as he had incredible faith in his words. I attempted once more and finally, after sixteen hours of going without, I drifted away to sleep.

Aftermath.

Gingerly, I woke up. A window covered the whole side wall. The sun glared brightly across the room and my bed. It was unusually hot. My mind was slowly coming to grips with what had occurred. I remembered the issue I had with my eyes and I realised that my pupils had returned to their normal state. They were still sore though from all the tension of being pulled to the side. Mum was sitting on a chair and she greeted me with a smile. I was still in ICU; my body felt like it had been beaten up. Rightly so, after a chaotic hour of injections, oxygen pumped into my system, fluids, heart rate going up, high blood pressure, eyes out of sync, tongue swelling up, throat clogged, dehydrated, unable to eat or drink, weariness due to lack of sleep and doctors/nurses trying to find out the cause and solution of the reaction. It was a big victory, a victory of faith over fear when my thoughts were betraying me. If it was not for Dad speaking into my ears, it may have been a different story. Fear easily would have swallowed me up, sapping my strength to fight. I thanked God for refreshing me with his words of assurance, confidence and affirmation while I was drowning in a sea of doubt. There really is incredible power of words spoken into your life.

My body cried out for some hydration and sustenance as I discerned that I had not eaten or drunk since before the whole ordeal. The nurse reminded me that I needed to fast for hours until my new catheter was surgically inserted into my underarm. Frustration overcame me. My body had endured this big hit from the anaphylactic attack. I had a new bone marrow finding its way into my bones. I was hot and sweaty because of the horrible sunlight that was shining through a window that was across the whole side of the room. Now I had to fast food and liquids until I had surgery. I felt like I was forced to go cold turkey, but was craving relief. I did not talk to the nurse out of protest to communicate my disdain for the situation. A frown painted itself on my face over the next few hours. Mum managed to sweet-talk the nurse into allowing me to have a cup of ice that I could slowly melt into my mouth. It was hard not to drink the whole cup of ice in one go as that was the only liquid I had access to over the next few hours. I needed to let it marinate in my mouth as long as I possibly could. Every hour, someone from the medical team would inform me that I would be in the surgery room within an hour, only for it to be delayed. This happened eight times. The sun was shining its rays right through the curtain-less, clean glass onto my bed as if it was mocking me, torturing me. This was a tough day to endure. This was not how I thought my first day of the bone marrow transplant would pan out. Finally, after twenty-four hours of fasting, a nurse informed me that we were finally going to go into surgery. There was a mini-celebration as I dreamt about the awful hospital food tasting like a sweet sensation of heaven after this surgery. It signalled a close to the horrible, 'foodless' aftermath. Surely everything was on the up from here.

Doubting the Process.

In the process so far, I had achieved a significant amount. I had completed two rounds of chemotherapy, received the bone marrow transplant, overcome a dangerous anaphylactic reaction, and the catheter had been re-inserted. My body was feeling the lingering effects of sickness. I felt the aches everywhere, as well as the fumes of the aches. It was a double whammy. I had headaches, muscle aches, tummy aches, sore throat, gastro, no appetite, nor any energy. My drive and vision was dwindling every day as I was reminded by my body how sick I was. My focus was all on the issue at hand. Doubt was becoming a regular visitor once again, bringing negativity into my mind. As a result, I began to question God's work in me. It was hard to see any increase in my health as progress, if any was made, was going slow. Dad continued to be a regular presence throughout my nights since I had the reaction to ensure that I was safe and okay. I continually asked him one question daily: *how long will it take for me to recover?* I needed assurance that I was on the right track. Dad would always answer the same way. *It might be soon, or it might be a long time. Everyone is different. Just keep pushing through.* It was a different predicament for me because my strength could be my weakness. My strength often made me feel independent, for I did not ask for God's help. So far in life, my strength and health had been a real asset in my life. I never really needed God (according to me) in that area of life. I had always been ready to fight, been strong in mind and passion, been fit and active; always seeking to participate. Now, my health was stripped away, my strength sapped. It made me feel vulnerable. Because of this diagnosis, I ran to God for help. I needed to rely on God to be my source of strength, my beacon of hope because he is faithful to the promises he has made. Yet, here I was, in the deep end of the pool, struggling to float and now doubting whether God really was who he was cracked up to be.

The water was bubbling up above my head and suffocating my breath. I was struggling to see if the lifeguard was coming to save me. Doubt continued to feed my mind. I quickly shook it off and remembered what I said to God—*Even when it looks bad. I will trust you.* I could not see

God around, but I decide to hold onto these words to help me through. Meanwhile, Doubt reclined back into his chair, plotting his next words; not wanting to squander his second opportunity with me.

Weary.

Two weeks passed by since the bone marrow transplant. Every day was looking like the same day: lots of sleep, no progress, loss of motivation. God had disappeared. I was not hearing his voice or seeing him around. *He had left me in my toughest moments. How dare he?* My body was battered, bruised, shaken up as the procedure further took its toll. My strength was drained every single day, like a battery running out of juice. *Surely this is not sustainable? My health is meant to be increasing since the transplant! Yet I feel like I am going to croak any time soon.* Mum was about to check out and she looks at me intently. *Everything okay James?* I nod my head unconvincingly. Mum's intuition picks it up. She looked at me longer, waiting. I couldn't hold it any longer; my emotions bubble to the surface, my exterior cracked and I started crying uncontrollably. Mum moved quickly and hugged me. *I miss home! I miss school. I miss my friends. I miss doing things. I miss being around people. It just keeps getting worse. I keep trying to talk to God but I have not heard from him. I do not know what to do.* Everything I felt and think continued to pour out of my mouth. My frustrations, worries, burdens and fears blurted out in between deep sobs. Everything in the past three weeks had been building up weight and pushing me down further into the darkness. I felt like I was swimming against the tide, with no rest in sight. My attitude, mentality and strength were being seriously tested. I did not know if I could go any further. I wanted it all to stop. I was done. Mum held me in her arms as she tried to comfort me, knowing this situation was beyond our understanding. There was a sense of release after the emotional outpour, but I was still weak, burdened by the immensity of this battle. I did not know where I would find the extra ounce of faith that I needed to continue pushing. I was on the fringes of the cliff, waiting to fall off.

Peace.

After I came to grips with myself, letting all my emotions pour out, Mum finished up for the day and went home. The nurses were out of the room and I was alone. My illnesses and aches were amplifying in this moment. My body was feeling even more weary. There was no strength to draw from. I felt my body groaning louder and louder. I was in a daze, feeling every ache become worse, building to its tipping point. I shouted *Enough!* Instantly, all my illnesses vanished, my aches relieved. Pure silence overcame me. No thoughts, no voices, no noises. There was such pure silence that I could see the quietness. Peace. I took a few deep breaths and I heard God. *Now sleep.* I closed my eyes and fell asleep straight away. It was the most peaceful, dreamless, deepest sleep I have ever had in life. It was as if my body clocked off and shut down momentarily. I normally have nurses coming in throughout the night to complete their check-ups for me, but I did not remember one coming in throughout the night. Peace and sleep was all that I knew right now.

The morning after, I woke up and there was a freshness in the air; a different vibe that rang through. My mind caught up with what was happening and I noticed that I was still sick. My aches and symptoms remained, however I felt refreshed; my strength anew. I felt strong, despite what my body was going through. My mentality and attitude seemed to have recovered. I turned and noticed God was with me. He smiled at me. God knew I needed rest; a break from the sickness to help me recover my strength—physically, mentally, and emotionally. This newfound strength and drive provided a beacon of hope for me. I could get through this season. *Thank you God. I do not know what you did but I needed it.* God acknowledged it with a smile. *I was always here; I am always here. Sometimes I need to see how you respond when you think I am not.* I knew I was going to be okay now, especially since God relieved me of my suffering for one night. It paid huge dividends. I felt different now, stronger. God empowered me spiritually, strengthened me as I had faith and trust in him. With God, I was confident I had the victory. Without God, I was struggling to see the victory—especially with the circumstances and problems piling up and becoming overwhelming burdens. The amazing perk of having God as my friend is that I can cast my cares and worries to him, knowing full well that he can provide what I need. The stories must be true after all: God was still here with me, helping me fight. My faith in him continued to grow.

*

Revelation.

Three years after this moment, God provided me with a vision of a different perspective of the night he took away my sickness temporarily and told me to rest. *I am looking through the door, inward to the room I am staying in for the treatment, the Fish Bowl. I gaze through and see myself on the hospital bed. Struggling, groaning, and turning. To the right of the bed, I see a spirit-like figure walk across, inching closer to my bed. The spirit-like figure turns to me and immerses itself into my body and disappears. I am taken aback, as I attempt to make sense of what is occurring. I look at myself again and I see myself overwhelmed with peace. I realize that God's spirit has taken my place for the night, taking what my sickness, illness, and aches. So I can rest, recuperate, and regain my strength again. I stand back, awestruck, marvelling at the power and care of God.*

It is at this moment that I knew God would not give me more than what I could handle. It felt that sometimes I was overwhelmed by what was going on, but God knew I could push through it. I would be stretched, but the promise from God was that I would not break. As I was stretching in these tough circumstances, I was increasing in strength, endurance, perseverance, trust, and ultimately, faith. This was a revelation that I held onto daily. I could overcome what was coming my way and if not, God would provide the necessary tools for me to do so.

*

Lazy.

After regaining my strength, yet still carrying aches; I felt a mixture of determination, apathy and laziness; an understanding that I still needed to work to push through this, but a yearning to go home and be done with it. As I had been bedridden for days, sleeping extremely long hours, my body had adjusted to this lazy regime. My doctor barged in the room with her team behind her and opened all the blinds across the window side to let the sunlight shine through, despite my protest. *James needs to start doing things and staying awake if he wants to recover.* My mum got the message and agreed. My parents began forcing me to get out of bed everyday into the shower. It was hard to do so because it meant I had to get out of my comfortable bed and move around more than I had those past weeks, despite my stomach ache and sore muscles. I would have rather stayed in a smelly bed if it meant I did not become uncomfortable. It was fascinating how one chore that I easily did every day for my own hygiene became so hard and something I dreaded to initiate. Like clockwork, every morning, Dad would tell me to get out of bed and have a shower. I grumbled and stated that I felt unwell. Each time they will threw me this line—*If you do not get out of bed and have a shower, you will never get better.* They knew my desire to get better was the trump card for me. It was simply the matter of feeding this motivation to help me gain the strength to get up and moving. I always felt better instantly after my shower. The sensation of hot water streaming down my body felt as though it was cleansing me of my illness. It became a time of enjoyment; allowing the heat and water distracted me from my physical illnesses, helped me ponder deep thoughts. It was another escape for me. Each morning I got up to go to the shower, it became *slightly* easier to do so the next morning. It was the little things that I did daily which brought my prayer for a speedy recovery closer and reachable.

Physiotherapist.

Since my anaphylactic reaction from the chemotherapy, I developed pneumonia, which caused breathing difficulties in my lungs, which is a potential side effect of going through this treatment. A physiotherapist became part of my team to assist me on the road to recovery. She had the hardest job. She was my enemy and my best friend. I did not want to do any exercise. I wanted to do nothing but sleep my way through it all. Her role was to help me build up my lung capacity once again, help my breathing issues, and ultimately assist me to become my fit and active self once again. Every day, at three o'clock, she would come in. Before that, every day, I turned to my Mum and said *I am really tired and exhausted, please do not wake me up for the next hour or so, under any circumstances.* I closed my eyes and the physiotherapist arrived shortly after. I slightly opened my eyes to observe the scene. She greeted my mum with a smile and generated a little small talk about how I was travelling. Mum informed her that today (like every other day) I was very tired. She responded with a sympathetic *Aww*; then jumped straight to me yelling, *alright! Get up James and let us do our exercises for today.* My plan never ever worked; it was always foiled. Bitterness eroded within my heart. She was crazily determined to get me up and moving; which did not bode well for someone who wanted to be lazy and do absolutely squat.

I began with a horrible breathing exercise. I had this equipment where I needed to breath as hard and long as I could, pushing the little ball as high I could and then had to repeat it thirty times. It took every ounce of energy and breath to complete this exercise. I was rendered to exhaustion. It did nothing for my mental drive. I felt like I had completed a marathon and just wanted to drop and die. After this, she would make me get out of bed and get my legs moving on a bike-like pedal machine. I always refused, but she ended up compromising by telling me to only do twenty seconds of it. I placed my feet and did one circular motion on it and instantly rolled back to bed. She never gave up and got me back up again. She urged me to do two minutes worth of exercise, then she would leave me alone. I grumbled and slowly moved the pedals. If I had to do two minutes, I would milk it as slowly as I could. She hit me with a barrage of motivation words. I felt seething anger from the bitterness of her making me do work rising up within my body; burning passion that built up from her annoying insistence to exercise. I went slightly faster as a result. *I do not want to exercise. I want to sleep. No one ruins my sleep and gets away with it. I do not like you.* She responded with a big grin as I was pedalling faster than ever before. *Good James. Good! Use that anger and keep going.* Her joy in my anger made be angrier because my message was not being communicated. As I was seething with anger, my legs were pummelling wildly on the pedal machine. Before I knew it, I was finished and she was satisfied with my workout regime for the day. Until tomorrow... I went back to back filthy at the emotion I am wearing, but satisfied that I had put in the work that would help me get better.

Comparison.

The weeks were passing by; the homesickness was growing. I wanted to go back home to my family and friends and live out a social life with freedom. I wanted to play, have fun and enjoy life. Mum kept me updated with the other patients in the other rooms as the mums collectively shared what was happening with their kids and provided support for one another. There were four isolated rooms in the ward that the hospital called 'The Fishbowl'. I was in the third room. There was another boy, same age as me, who had come in after I did. He needed a stem cell transplant; different procedure to mine but same kind of illness as me. From what I heard, he seemed worse off than me. I felt slightly encouraged at the thought of this. *I am not doing as bad as I could be.* Before I knew it, I heard that the transplant was so successful. The boy was eating like a machine, working out and his health was rapidly increasing. Comparing myself to him built doubt and frustration within me. I was barely eating, unable to find the motivation to move and having slow progress in my health. He ended up getting the permission to leave after a two-week stay, while I was toiling in my fourth week! As good as it was to hear good news for a boy I never met, it was difficult for me to absorb the news. It caused me to question my own ability to recover from this.

Hard Yards.

My mentality began to shift when it came to approaching hard work to help me get better. It was amazing how I wanted things, yet I was currently not prepared to do the hard work. I was meant to be partnering with God in this process, but he was not going to do it all for me while I lay passive. I couldn't do what God was doing, and God certainly would not do my part because that responsibility laid with me. God reminded me that I needed to be diligent and hard-working if I wanted to see something good come out of this. He reminded me of the verse, Colossians 3:23 - *Whatever you do, work heartily, as for the Lord and not for men.* How could I expect God to fulfil my prayers and promises if I was slacking off, hoping for God to do it all? It took time, toil and work before I could expect God to rain down his promises.

There is a quote from the movie *"Facing the Giants"* which resonated with me at this point.

"Grant, I heard a story about two farmers who desperately needed rain. And both of them prayed for rain, but only one of them went out and prepared his fields to receive it. Which one do you think trusted God to send the rain?"

"Well, the one who prepared his fields for it."

"Which one are you?" Mr. Bridges continued. "God will send the rain when He's ready. You need to prepare your field to receive it."

This was an amazing rhetorical question for me. It held a simple answer. If I was to believe God would initiate a speedy recovery, allowing my story to inspire and reach out to the magnitude of people that I envisioned, I needed to do my hard yards. I trusted God during an anaphylactic attack, cried out to him. I felt sick and ready to stop. I had to put in work in showering every day, staying awake as long as I possibly could, exercising as much as I could, studying and reading to strengthen my mind, eating when my stomach wanted none of it. I couldn't do anything to eradicate the cancer, or boost my immune system to overcome it. I could pray. I could work on my body to stay healthy and well. God provided me with the key idea I need to hold onto in the season ahead. *I need to stop sitting around, only praying; but pray and doing what I need to do in anticipation and preparation for the answer to come.*

Progress.

November 3rd 2010. I hit a significant milestone in the recovery process. My white blood cells finally increased to the appropriate number to enable me to take a small walk outside my fishbowl (into another small, enclosed room next door). It seemed little, but it was a huge step; the first time I was out of the room in five weeks. I stepped out of my isolation room and outside the four walls I had been contained in. I looked at Mum and smiled. *It smells different.* Mum was amused. I walked around, slow-paced, for five minutes. Afterwards, I ventured back into my room and rested. As soon as I sat down, my body just threw up uncontrollably. I could not believe that my body reacted so badly after a simple task. I was happy, however, because I felt my body was beginning the process of adapting to walk again. It was ridding itself of the bad contents, allowing it to be easier when I walked next time. Every hurdle I jump over was one less hurdle I had to overcome and one step closer to the finish line.

Breakthrough

November 8th, 2010. An excited nurse walked into the room with incredible news. She announced that I was going home in the evening. Dad became concerned that it was a false alarm, getting my hopes up for nothing. I shrugged it off and believed the nurse. She was true to her word and prepped me to go home that night. The nurse was in my room and gave me a summary of all the tablets and pills that I needed to take and the different times of the day they needed to be taken. There was a mammoth amount of pills, all different sizes: big and small, all different colours. One was as big as a peanut! There were twelve pills to be taken, some around two to four times a day. I felt sick at the thought of this; seeing all the different textures, colours and flavours. I stepped on the scales to weigh myself. I was fifty-two kilograms. I weighed sixty-two before I came in. I had lost ten kilograms, mostly leg strength after lying in bed all that time. I received the last of my fluids, the final warnings from the doctor and complimentary hugs from the nurse as they saw one of their own flock leaving.

Steps.

It was a wonderful sensation walking out of the 'fishbowl'. There was a sense of unknown danger lying ahead, yet a complete trust in God. Mum began to feel nervous as she felt the weight of looking after me upon her shoulders. My facemask was on to limit and prevent any germs invading my fragile body. I walked through the hospital and there was a flight of six steps. Naturally, I made my way, up but as soon as I stepped onto the second step, my legs practically gave way. My body leaned back, nearly falling. I grabbed the railing and found my footing on the bottom of the steps again. I laughed at myself as Mum tried to figure out why I was still at the bottom of the steps. I marvelled at how my muscles had become so relaxed and loose during the time of rest and lack of exercise. I felt ridiculous, thinking that I couldn't walk up a short flight of steps. It hit me: *I still have a long way to go.* With a concerted effort and support from

Mum; I walked up the stairs. A feeling of accomplishment overcame me. No mountain, big or small, was going to stop me from succeeding this challenge.

Home.

There was incredible nostalgia as I arrived home, seeing a tidy house, a clean bedroom. Familiar sights triggered feelings of comfort and security. I saw my dogs in the distance, wagging their tails in excitement, but unable to make contact with them because of my low immunity. I had defeated, possibly, the toughest part of this battle. This stage was all about recovering and persevering towards the goal. The most difficult point of this stage was walking in the unknown. There could be any setback that could come my way if I was not careful. Although I hold onto one constant: God. It was hard making decisions, goals, finding motivation, when the path ahead was unpredictable. Anything could happen in regards to the transplant. I could become sick anytime, have a reaction, a side effect could arise, or the bone marrow may have failed in my system. This sense of unpredictability was testing my trust in God. It was taking a lot of faith to believe in the promises that God had made; that I would actually achieve the goals I set before myself. I ensured that I had the focus of trusting God as the solid rock for me to stand on.

Goals.

The sense of unpredictability was really testing my trust in God. The motivation was wavering as I fluctuated between doubt and belief in the process as I kept looking at the mountain hovering over me. I knew I could keep going, but it was the hard work ahead that needed to be done calling for me to quit. I needed to do this for myself, for God, and for the people ahead to be astonished at what had occurred. I began writing down five goals that I would achieve in order to put something in stone; something I could look at, use as a measuring stick, and draw motivation from. I wrote down these five goals and publicly shared them.

1. I would fully recover by March (or earlier)
2. I would be back at my high school in Year 12, sometime during term 1 (or even from the start)
3. I would be back playing basketball by April
4. I would compete in the Sports Tradition at my school—The Windsor Gardens Exchange
5. God would initiate a speedy recovery so that the world would see God's glory in my battle

As it was shared publicly, it was met with various responses. Some were cheering me on, applauding my strength; others were doubting whether it was a good idea to have those goals when I should put my health first. As unpredictable everything was, it was made harder by the doubters around me. Bless their heart; I am sure they had good intentions of looking out for me, concerned that I was setting myself up for setbacks, failures and/or disappointment. However, it only fuelled my motivation. My whole life, I have had to prove people wrong, prove myself, and in doing so, have pushed myself to greater lengths. Whenever someone questioned whether I could do something, it became a challenge that I wanted to rise to. My doctor heard that I wanted to be back at school, doing year twelve within a few months. She completely rejected the idea, saying *there was no chance. It is not realistic. You will not be back at school until Term two, and even then, it will not be a full load.* As a doctor in charge of my progress, it was a hit for my belief in this goal. It nearly shut the door of opportunity for God to move within my situation. My fire to succeed became bigger. I put those words on the back of my mind and decided to keep focusing on God and the goals I have set. In order to achieve this, I needed to look after myself well, train my body to become stronger and healthier. Losing ten kilograms has caused my body to be a weak and slim frame. I needed to rebuild my body, strengthen my muscles and get back into better shape than ever before. I looked at the mountain hovering over me. I smiled. I began walking up towards the summit with a fierce determination not to be defeated.

Education.

As I was now at home, recovering in isolation and the school year was beginning in two months, there were conversations happening around my schooling future and the best option. The main issue everything hinged on was how well I recover and the best way to work education around it. I had been completing homework via correspondence from my school teachers until I stopped closer to my transplant; understandably because I lacked motivation, brain power, health and had bigger things to worry about. Doing so meant I had missed out on two months of schoolwork in year eleven. The homework had piled up itself and felt like a huge burden every time I looked at it. It was something I was told to do in my own time when I felt like it. Not the best way to motivate a student! As my family and teachers discussed the best opportunities for me in regards to schooling and the circumstances of my recovery, mentality, and being in isolation, they came up with five different options.

1. Do distance education for year 12
2. Taking the year off
3. Do year 12 over 2 years
4. Drop out of school
5. Do Bible College earlier (My choice of post high school studies)

None of the options mentioned doing year twelve at my high school, graduating with the people I grew up in school with. It was tough as I had my heart set on it. The doctors and teachers were trying to give me the best option to further my education and give me the best position to advance in life and career. It was becoming hard to convince myself, let alone my teachers and doctors, to allow me to do year twelve. It was due to the fact that the main timeline for a person recovering from a bone marrow transplant is six to twelve months. If this remained true for me, then I would not be able to attend school till April at the bare minimum. It did not work because I would need an attendance record above ninety percent, which was physically impossible as I was not free from isolation yet.

Options.

I did not like the idea of doing Bible College earlier because I would have to do a Diploma before a Bachelor of Arts due to not finishing year twelve. I did not want to drop out of school because I really wanted to see through my commitment in school and place myself in the best position for life. I did not want to take the year off because I was driven and wanting to get the ball rolling to finish school. With all this in mind, the teachers claimed the best option was Distance Education, or do year twelve over two years. Alarm bells were sounding off in my head because my heart was stubbornly not letting go of the desire to complete the goal I set before myself. We had meeting after meeting with the school every time there was new progress in my health and further advancements in my decision for my schooling. The teachers and school board were amazing in sacrificing time to help me get the best opportunity for schooling. This thought was not lost on me. It was frustrating though that they tried to convince me, with good intentions, to take the opportunity they lay in front of me. Being driven to hold onto my goal, I did not budge. I was becoming frustrated because I felt that I was not being given the space to pursue what I strongly felt God has placed in my heart to do. There was tension between the best option and the God option. No one mentioned the God option of going straight back to school except for me. I wanted to attack with Plan A and jump into year twelve, succeeding. I began to wonder if it was all a pipedream. I questioned whether God really gave me the idea to do year twelve. If so, I did not want to settle for a measly option that would 'help' me, as it would forfeit God's plan in my situation. It was me and God against everyone else. The teachers were as frustrated as I was for I did not budge while I internalised this monologue within my mind.

At that point, it looked like I was going to have to do Distance Education for the first year of year twelve and then go back to school for the second year; completing year twelve over two years. I felt the struggle of trying to place my trust in God and to see the plan through while being pulled in the other direction of people saying the other option was the best way to go. I began to become influenced that it was possibly the best option because everyone kept telling me so. I was under immense pressure to press forward with this option, listening to the advice of others who believed so. I was still recovering, my mind was still not in its best shape and I was struggling to make a decision. It became a battle of conviction and natural sense. Was I to stand firm on the option I believed God had called me to take, which no one considered was working, or take the option which seemed to make sense? It was adding unnecessary stress to myself when I should have been focusing on getting better. I needed to plan and sort myself out for the short-term, and long-term, if I was going to choose to fight for one option, or go with the flow on the other option. I knew I need to talk to God. I had to ask him what he wanted me to do.

Inquire.

As I spoke with God, I did not get a specific answer to which option I should take, but I did get the sense that something was in the works. God reminded me of the story of King David. *Throughout King David's reign over Israel, David continually inquired me of what to do. He asked for advice, permission, guidance; and whatever answer he got, he obeys. Sometimes in life, you can get caught up in what is going on and end up following your own direction. Keep on inquiring of me and I will lead the way.* This recalibrated my focus onto God. I believed that God had told me what the option was already. I needed to hold onto it. I needed to continue to trust the source of my plan, to go back to God for guidance when I was unsure of my direction. Something was in the works, although I did not know what.

A few days later, I flicked through the paperwork for Distance Education to familiarise myself with the program, as it was presented as the best option for me. I scanned through the contents and something came to light. God drew my attention to something very small, but specific within the paperwork. I discovered that the Media class material was different to the material at my high school. I realized that it would be impossible to do half of a year with Distance Education and the other half at my high school when I was better in year twelve because it was different material for one full year. This was it. This was the clause I needed to know to avoid Distance Education as an option. The idea was either not do Distance Education, or commit fully to it, which I did not want to do. I ran to Mum and shared what I found. My mum understood there was a conflicting idea that would not allow me to transfer from Distance Education back to school with ease. We figured we would bring it up at the next school meeting, which was when the final decision was to be made. A mini victory for me!

Work.

In between this time and the meeting, there was something I had to do if I was to act on the belief that I would be back at school. It was homework; the big stack of sheets piled up on my desk, taunting me each time I walked past them. The idea that I may not even make it back at school made it harder for me to find motivation to do it. *What if I do the work, but it ends up being fruitless when I do not go back to school?* I thought at the time. I did not like the idea of doing work and motivation was a rare find during this time. I walked to Dad to share my lack of motivation. *Dad, if there is a chance I may not do year twelve, why waste my time to do homework? I said to him.* Dad responded with a question: *What does your faith tell you?* Instantly I knew the answer. *That I will do Year twelve.* Dad then assured me that I needed to do the work if I wanted to see God do the work in me. I needed to do my part and God would do his. I became overwhelmed with a renewed vigour and motivation to tackle the work. I hit the homework hard, frantically trying to do as much work as I could because the desire to complete my goals became huge. I marvelled at how I went from battling cancer to gaining motivation to complete schoolwork. God really was at work in me. I only needed to act on this faith knowledge and do the work beforehand; displaying that I truly believed what God wanted me to do.

Biopsy.

The development of my education options only became a finality once I got the results of my biopsy right before school began. The results painted a picture of what I could and could not do. It became hard to wait around for the date of my biopsy and the results. I wanted to know the progress I had made so far and whether I could go to school or not. In the lead up, I focused on what I could do, looking after myself: taking my tablets, drinking four litres of fluids a day, building up my body and appetite again, completing my homework. Despite not being certain that I would be at school soon, by faith, I put in the work.

January 12th 2011. The day of my biopsy arrived. It was exciting knowing that this operation would provide me with the answers, but nervousness crept in, as it would also provide the finite decision of whether I could do school or not. After I woke up from the biopsy, my first thoughts were of God. *I have done my bit, now do yours. It is your glory; choose what you want to do with it.* There was a sense of joy that I could not explain. It might have been the understanding that I had no control of anything, but God had control over everything and God was outworking the situation that was best for me. It was a lightweight burden as it was all in God's hands. I eagerly waited to let people know the results. I really wanted it to be an answer to what people had been praying for—a breakthrough.

Results.

January 31ˢᵗ 2011. We had a meeting with my doctor to discuss my biopsy results on how well my bone marrow was recovering and following this, we had a meeting with school to make a decision on my schooling future. School began in a few days, so it was a big day with many ramifications. I could easily feel rushed with the recovery and preparation for school, but I was in a calm state of mind, prepared in knowing that I had put the work in with my homework, strengthening my mind and energy. I walked into the meeting with my doctor with one burning question: *Could I go back to school?* She looked up my results and took a few moments to ponder. *James, I am happy with your progress,* she told me. *However, it is not one hundred percent.* I did not know what to make of that. I let the thought run through my mind for a moment. *So, can I go back to school or not?* She took a deep breath, filling me with dread momentarily. *At the end of the day, it is your choice. The less you do during this period, the less risk you have of setbacks with infections or sickness due to your recovering immunity.*

My mouth dropped in shock. I wanted to pinch myself. *Did she just say it is my choice? Did she just leave the onus onto me?* She had been authoritative and strict for my sake and benefit but now, she had given me the option. She was firm, but she gave me a little space for me to operate with. It was all I needed. A sense of optimism built within me. I was content and ready to see what unfolded at the school meeting. On the way out, I bumped into the teacher that helped me throughout my hospital stay. She had been well-informed of my situation and progress. She quickly asked what the outcome was for my schooling. With confidence, I bluntly shared, *I want to do year twelve full time this year. To do it all within one year.* The expression on her face said it all. There was doubt, shock and something communicating to me to be prepared for disappointment. *That is a big ask.* Tell me something I do not know. I continued to hold onto God's promise. The dominos were currently rolling my way so far. Conviction built up within me and I finished off by stating *we will get it one way or another.* She knew there was no changing my mind, so she gave me her well-wishes for the meeting.

Meeting.

A few hours later, my parents and I walked into the meeting ready to decide on an outcome for my situation. My family was wanting the best outcome for me that would hold me in the best stead, like any other loving parent, but I was firm on which outcome I desired. The opening of the meeting consisted of the results of the biopsy. My parents shared that the bone marrow was progressing very well, although I was not completely recovered in my immune system. I shared the issue of Distance Education program and the predicament it had put me in; either do it completely or not at all. The staff understood and let it saturate in their minds. I put forth my desire to do year twelve at this high school. This limited the options we had after all the weeks of discussing and researching. With good intentions, the staff voiced their concern of me becoming unwell again if I did push myself to go straight back to school within a few days. It was a barrier they struggled to move pass: putting my well-being at centre stage. They pushed back with the option of doing it part-time over two years.

I knew I needed to come to a decision quickly because the teachers were concerned by the natural circumstances—results, risk, and the reality of the situation—whereas I was focusing on God's promise for me. It was a risky situation, but I needed to make a bold step of faith. I responded with conviction and a firm tone: *I really want to do school over one year and graduate with my friends.* Again, they pushed back with more concerns. The teachers shared the 'what if' situations. *What if you get sick again? What if you end up becoming worse?* The 'what ifs' presented doubt in my mind. I understood their point, but it was make or break for me. This was the final meeting we had. God planted an idea in my mind: that I needed to take full responsibility for myself. I respond. *If I get sick again, I have to deal with that. I will drop out and deal with the setback, failing my comeback bid. On the other hand, if I do not get sick again, I complete what I want to achieve. At the end of the day, it is on me. Whatever happens to me, I accept full responsibility for. It is all or nothing.* The teachers all layed back in their chairs, as they saw an epitome of conviction before their eyes. They looked at each other with an unspoken sense of agreement. They knew I was committed and that if anyone could push through it, I could. To my delight, they all came to an agreement and allowed me to attempt to finish my final year of school. What an incredible result.

The staff even went an extra step further and began placing a framework and boundaries for me to have in the first couple of weeks so they could limit the risk of me becoming sick again while my immunity recovered. The framework created was that I was in class for two subjects and out of class for my other two subjects. They provided a room (nicknamed 'The Box') for me near the theatre rooms for me to complete work by myself via correspondence. The teachers offered to come around every now and then to assist me with my questions. I was only to be around a small group of friends for the time being and not attend assembly, which the whole school assembled for. I marvelled at the ease of the plan the teachers created for me and their willingness to support me after being so hesitant to commit to my desired outcome. It was amazing that God's plan was in activation after months of debating, setbacks and working through it. I was able to snowball the momentum of building and displaying my faith in God after the intense hospital stay. I had the breakthrough, now came the follow-through. I needed to put in more work to see the incredible story come to pass of what God was doing in my life ever since I approached him to get to know him. The greater the challenges, the greater the victory. School started in three days. I did not know how it was going to turn out, but I was ready to walk through it.

Seed.

With every breakthrough in life, there comes a need for a follow-through—whether it comes in the form of carrying out a promise after receiving an opportunity in life, performing your role after breaking through a barrier, or simply maintaining a standard after pushing for so long and hard for progress. Even though I had finally overcome my stay at the hospital, my darkest hours being sick, and the barriers in trying to resume my education, I still had to match my words and put in the hard work to complete my education, all whilst attempting to remain healthy. The battle was not over yet; it was not going to be easy. Anything could happen to try and derail me. It was not a time to lower my guard down, but to continue with my follow-through to see this challenge to the very end. I was back at school, but it was not without its challenges. It is funny to look back on, but I would pray for a tree, but get annoyed at God when he provided me with the seed for the tree. I would love to have a complete recovery and ultimate freedom to do what I wanted to do in school, but there was no growth in that. God reminded me that life was about growing, persevering and conquering.

God had given me enough to operate with and I still faced the challenge of getting myself into shape. My mind was still mush after not being engaged in learning and being challenged. My mind needed to be sharpened once again to face the regime of school so quickly after enduring chemotherapy and a bone marrow transplant. I decided to do the one thing I could do: stick my head down and work hard through it all, while trusting that God was going to help grow the seed. A noticeable blessing was that I had nearly all the same teachers from my previous year, bar one. This meant the teachers were aware of my situation, and understood what I was capable of. This enabled the teachers to know how to best teach me, when to push my limits, and when to hold back, letting me be. For the first few weeks, I was able to complete the schoolwork given to me, although I knew it was not my best work due to my brain still developing its prowess of doing work. Each day I was at school, I was getting better and better, slowly growing into the mould of what I had committed to do.

Sometimes I felt like I had a brand new body, as I was still testing out the muscles that had been unused for months. The first time I ran, my muscles cramped up in my calves and I couldn't walk for three days. I kicked a football for the first time and I pulled a hamstring. My body was in mint, fragile condition! It was a challenge to face my boundaries at school because I wanted to run out and celebrate with my fellow students that I was back, yet I had to be disciplined, under the watchful eye of staff, being careful not to put myself in any precarious situation.

Risk.

I decided I had had enough of being in the small room, the Box and I was getting annoyed in not being able to participate with the other students. There was an assembly occurring and I decided to inquire to God whether I ought to try something. I felt a pull to go into the building where the school was having an assembly. The boundaries stated I was not to do so, but I felt a tug within my heart. *You will keep me protected, won't you God?* I felt a sense of assurance and made my move. I wandered casually into the foyer. Soon, a rush of students came through. Six hundred students walked past me. The ones that knew me were surprised and gave me their smiles and greetings. Eventually, one of the teachers saw me in the foyer and was met with shock. Looking out for me, she consoled me and made sure I was sent back to my room. I walked back to the box, hidden away from the chaos and flocks of students. In the aftermath, I was met with annoyed teachers, throwing their arms up as to why I was willing to risk it by walking into the assembly. My parents heard about it and questioned my motives. I told them that I felt like doing it. Deep down, I used the situation as a testament of my faith, holding God to his promise that he would protect me (within his command) and I would not become sick from the experience. Every now and then, a teacher would remind me of my stupidity and shake their head, unable to understand why I walked into the assembly. They could only see the small picture; the surface level of what I was doing.

Pills

Throughout this period, I was still on a truckload of pills and tablets, to be taken at all sorts of hours in my day. I began to get sick of these pills; my body groaned at the thought of taking pills. I began to debate whether I could get away with taking less, or missing out on a few. The texture of the pills was causing me to feel sick. It was like eating Brussel sprouts throughout my day. I was sick of it. I asked God again, *is it okay if I do not take these pills? Will you protect me?* I heard no response stopping me, so I decided to skip a few pills. A few pills become a lot of pills. A lot of pills became all the pills. Eventually I was not taking anything, with no one noticing. It was risky, but I was done with it. Here was hoping that it paid off.

Sleep.

A dominant aspect of my routine was sleep. I had 'free' periods', or 'study' periods, as my teachers liked to emphasize. It was in those times that I was able to sleep. My body was not yet adapting to working hard mentally or being awake for a full twelve-hour day. Throughout my schedule, I needed to refresh and recover hourly. Every moment I could find, I ended up napping. I slept in my free periods in the Box, probably the most advantageous reason to be in my own room and blocking myself from all the external noise. I slept sometimes during lunch. I slept when I got home, on the carpet, on my bed, wherever I could find. It was incredible how I could find time and places to sleep and have a mini-recovery session without being disturbed or worrying about anyone annoying me. This enabled me to get through my day somewhat strongly and work towards my goal of recovering fully and completing year twelve by the end of that year.

April.

April, 2011. The holidays came around and I had completed my first term of schooling. The defining month had arrived; the month that I declared that I would be fully recovered by. I had my biopsy during the holidays and now awaited my results. Before I found out, there was a conference that I could attend. Hundreds of Christians flocked to this conference and I really wanted to go, but I did not have the full clearance yet. I wanted to take another step of faith and risk it to believe that I was healed, despite not knowing the results. By now, I had a hefty head of hair full of curls. I wanted to get a haircut to look somewhat presentable in public, but God placed a thought into Mum's mind: *Samson*. Samson is a man whose hair gave him incredible strength. Knowing that I wanted to go to the conference, Mum placed incredible faith in God and this thought—*What if you do not shave your head, and God gives you the strength and protection to go to the conference? Especially after you spoke about Samson when you lost your hair…*It made sense to me. I was more bewildered that Mum was allowing me to go. God really must be at work! There was significance in this thought; I took the step of faith and attended the conference. There was not fear within me, nor doubt walking alongside me. I believed that I would not pick up a virus or anything that would trigger my sickness again. God was walking alongside me, holding me under his protection.

Throughout the few days, I was reconnecting with the people from my church and youth, whom have been following my journey over the months. It was exciting to be greeted with such warmth and love by those I knew and missed. There was one thing I did pick up, however. I had been absent from these people for months and I was struggling to get into the rhythm of their conversations. It was as if life has moved on without me in those months and I was struggling to catch up. I shared these concerns to my friend. She shared supportive words and encouraged me to allow this season to take its time; to allow myself to become accustomed to the fact that I was back, and that I had been away for a few months. After the conversation, the perspective was so much better. I had too higher standards in my comeback. The best news was that after the conference, I was still healthy. Every faith step I had taken so far with God was paying off. My trust in God was growing.

Appointment.

A few days after the conference, I had my appointment with my Doctor about the latest biopsy results. I walked into the office. The Doctor greeted me and typed away, giving away nothing to me. I shifted in my seat, knowing I was so close to hearing an answer, but the unknown made me uncomfortable. I had taken so many risks these past few months that I wanted it to work out! The doctor looked at the monitor, reading my results. She turned to me with a smile.

You are all good!

My mind failed to fully comprehend what exactly she was communicating. I asked her to elaborate a little more.

You are fully recovered. Your immunity is right up where it needs to be and there are no issues or complications.

I was hit with utter shock and relief. I did not prepare myself to hear those words. I cannot describe how I was feeling or what I was thinking. In fact, my mind was empty, struggling to comprehend the greatest news I could receive at this point. Mum looked at me with a smile and a shock at the news as well. I had completed the transplant and the recovery. I was not restricted to isolation conditions anymore. *I WAS FREE.* I knew I still had to be careful, still had appointments to attend, and that I would have these battle scars to carry, but the worst was over. It was only onwards and upwards from here. Joy swelled up within me. No words can match the feeling, so I sat there soaking in the emotion, content. After the appointment, Mum and I made our way to the car with a sense of excitement. No words were exchanged between us, except *Praise God* as we both continued to work our head around what had just

96

happened. I plugged in my phone to the music player and my songs were on shuffle. Ironically enough, the first random song that was played was "Healer". I smiled at God, for I knew the song was no coincidence, but was impeccable timing. I sang the song in thankfulness and in worship for all he had done. There was a sense of fulfilment within me, yet an awareness that there was a season of work to be done with my schooling. One main thought stuck within my mind—*I have defeated cancer, I can do anything with God.*

Basketball.

After a six-month absence from one of my biggest passions, playing basketball, I desperately wanted to get back onto the court. I was calling up teams to see if they needed a player, but I had missed the deadline and every squad was practically full. Being as determined as I am, I decided to take a different route and look into forming my own team. I asked around a few friends who I knew enjoyed basketball. To my surprise, I was able to gather seven players and found an empty spot in the league, even though it was a little above our skill levels. I only wanted to play ball. My first game was approaching and I could not contain my excitement, especially to check another milestone off my goals list—*to play basketball by April.* We were up against a team called 'Puzzle' and it became one of the most horrible shooting performances I have been a part of because we were all learning how to play with each other and I was trying to get back into the groove of things. However, the most incredible part was I was expecting to be tired and panting five minutes into the game; instead I kept running, and running, and running. Before I knew it, the game was over and I had finished the game, feeling like I could go back out right again. I marvelled at how my body was already adapting to a high intensity workout. It reflected the hard work I had put in to get back into shape, to build up my body and to increase my fitness. Things were slowly shifting back into gear. I was at school, playing basketball and recovered. There was nostalgia surrounding me everywhere I went. I no longer had to dream about doing things anymore. I was living it.

Setback.

As part of my studies, I was participating in a financial services course at a bank to give me experience. It was a struggle, as I was way in over my head in this course. On this particular day, I was finding myself itchy, especially at my elbow. The whole day, I was scratching away. I did not pay particular attention as to why. I arrived home and I discovered that I had a massive rash across my elbow and arm. Initially, I panicked and I ran to my parents. Mum's first thought was that I had shingles, a painful version of chicken pox, which is expected after the transplant as my immunity had reset. Dad quickly reacted and decided to take me back to the hospital. Before we left the house, Dad prayed for protection over me. We drove off together. *God, do not have me work this hard, come this far, only to fall short of the goal.* My mind flicked between fear and faith. I could see this circumstance unfolding before me with great intimidation, yet I knew God had never failed me yet, so why start now? I was scared because anything can happen post-transplant, yet I knew God was not going to do all this work, only to have it go to waste. Dad comforted me and assured me that through God's strength, I would be okay. My brain rummaged through different thoughts, trying to work out what was going on and what would happen; perks of being an over-thinker.

I was in silence, knowing that I couldn't do anything but trust in God and see the outcome through. Messages were sent out by my family for prayers that my report would be good. The familiar prayer blanket once again clothed over me and I felt safer within the security of God. I arrived at the Emergency Department and Dad handed over the pre-written procedure established by my medical staff of what needed to happen if this scenario occurred. The medical team in the ward acted quickly and began assessing and examining me, eliminating what the causes may be to zero in what was happening. They continually asked me how I was. Each time I responded, *I am tired.* I laid on the bed, attempting to sleep as much as I could, trusting in the process of the medical staff. It was 10.00 p.m. and I had school the next day. I was exhausted. A doctor finally came in and shared the diagnosis. I had an unspecific allergy reaction called hives. All I needed was a type of liquid antibiotic and I would be fine. Relief overcame me. At least it was not anything drastic and I could continue moving forward to my goal. It was great to see how well myself and the family responded in this situation by trusting in God, despite the fear of what may have unfolded. Faith was being sharpened in every circumstance that passed by. God was doing work within us, moulding our hearts and building our faith in him.

I was back at school the next day as if nothing happened. The only evidence was that I was tired and my eyes were supported by black bags. I was able to push through and get through the day, showing phenomenal strength, driven by my motivation as God propelled me forward.

Baptism.

May 2011. A significant day had approached. I was committing to being baptized with my sister after situations prolonged it—being in hospital, sister being overseas. It felt that it was the perfect timing though. I look back and I see the tremendous growth of my faith, trust, and depth of my relationship with God that was crafted from the situations I had been through. This was a public declaration of who I was living life for: God. I first made a decision to give my life to God to see what he would do with it. Since then, God had built brick upon brick. It was only fair that I continued to live for God because God has done his end of the deal and was continuing to do so. Moments before the baptism, my pastor shared some words of encouragement and spoke specifically into each individual who was about to be baptized. He happily shared his encouragement to me. He shared that this was the closing of the previous chapter of my sickness, and the opening of a new chapter that God had in store for me. It rang true to my life at this point because that morning, I had a dream that conveyed meaning. *There are two hands, the left hand opens, with the palm facing upwards. The right hand remains as a closed fist. Placed on the left hand is a small red object. I observe it but I need some time to work out what it is. Soon I come to the conclusion that it is a red blood cell. The left hand becomes closed and crushes the cell. The left hand opens up again, showing the evidence of the disappearance of the cell. It closes again and turns downwards. My attention turns to the other fist and it is turning upward, slowly revealing what is in the other hand. Building up the anticipation and expectation, my heart skips at the suspense of discovery but I wake up and am left hanging.*

Despite not finding out, I knew that what mattered was that the chapter of sickness was closed and I was cured. I was looking forward to what God had in store for me, but I needed to keep my focus on Him and not on what was in the hand. It would be revealed to me as I lived out my journey with God. Soon after, I made the step of being baptized, with my family and church looking on, followed by a rousing applause and celebration. This was a decision that I was going to be living onwards from, a decision to remain in a relationship with God, who is more than an incredible friend to me.

Grind.

Over the months, I was having to push myself through my studies; head down, working hard till it was over. I was in a steady routine, plodding away in school day by day. Motivation was hard to come by these days, as it was slowly being drained by the work, like every other student. Schoolwork, essays and assignments were still being achieved one by one. My only source of achievement was, knowing that each day passing by was one day I did not have to do again, for it was my final year of schooling. As the holidays arrived, the teachers distributed a stack of homework for us to keep the ball rolling and keep our minds sharp. However, the issue was that each time I scraped to a holiday, my brain was fried and I was exhausted because the immense workload was a lot for my fragile mind. I used the holidays to rest, recuperate and restore my energy by doing nothing. I did not touch one page of homework assigned because I could not bear the thought of it. Looking after myself was the number one priority. It was funny though: each time the first day of school rolled around, I was in a massive rush, frantically completing all my homework in the first couple of days without getting noticed that I did not do my homework. Maybe God was looking out for me in more ways than one. In those months, I was loving basketball as it provided a fresh escape of the grind, building back up to my form and beyond. I continued to have regular monthly appointments with my doctor, who was monitoring my progress, giving me new vaccinations for my newly rebooted immune system. You could see the doctor was consistently pleased, although she maintained a professional outlook.

Misunderstanding.

As I was participating in the Financial Services Course, I was discovering that I was quite in over my head, especially after recovering from my hospital stay. It was hurting my motivation and enjoyment. I was learning that finance was not currently my area of passion. I was ending up back at school, fatigued and tired. I spoke about it with a staff member, but she pressured me to keep participating because it was a good opportunity. I felt like I was not being heard and was forced to continue. It got to the point where my productiveness was seriously low and my boss took notice. He gave me a little 'spray', which was well deserved and told me that I needed to step it up. I am glad that he did so as it gave me the courage to speak to him and let him know the reason for my unproductiveness—my lack of enjoyment. My boss was very surprised at the fact that I was not enjoying it and even more surprised at the pressure of someone telling me that I needed to keep going with this course. He was happy to let me go, as it was not working out for both of us. We thanked each other and parted ways. A burden was lifted off my shoulders and I felt much better for it. I could put all my focus wholly into my studies and the goal of finishing school. The next day, I was in the Careers Pathway Office, as I was called in by the Careers Counselor. She questioned my decision of dropping the course and I stated that it was for my own well-being and that I was not getting what I was meant to be getting out of it. The reason she threw a fit was because of the decision I had made. I would now get a 'fail' on my report, which meant I would not be able to complete my final year. Zero chance of passing. The thought hit me like a 'ton of bricks': *Did I just derail my whole progress of schooling because of one decision to not keep going with a course not part of school?* I felt compromised and vulnerable. I was shattered because I had come this far and was not enjoying one aspect of schooling so I chose to rid of it, yet it had caused me to fail. I was upset, angry and confused as to how I should have felt. It was made clear to me that I couldn't pass year twelve anymore, but I did not want to walk back into that bank and continue the course.

I questioned my careers counselor to make sure I had heard right and that there was no other way to pass or make amends. She gave me the one and only option—*go back and complete the course, or fail.* I walked away from the office frustrated. That night, I unloaded on my parents the issue that I was facing. It felt like a crisis; I did not want to fall short of my goal.

Ramification.

The very next day, I was called into another meeting with the other staff who were looking after me: two assistant principals, one who has followed my journey for the last six years, and another whom does not know me well. They had heard about the situation. I assumed that the Careers Counselor had spoken to them and that Dad also called in to query what was going on. They wanted to clarify the situation for me. I was feeling broken and neutral after the adrenaline rush of emotions yesterday. Professionally, the assistant principal lays down the criteria of passing year twelve. She stated that I needed to pass a minimum of four subjects in order to complete the year successfully. I was currently doing five, including the course. If I was to drop the course, I would not have a 'safety' pillow, meaning I needed to pass every subject I was doing for the year. She shared that as long as I passed all four subjects, I would be fine. This brought a huge relief to my mind. This was what I thought in the first place and the reason why I felt I could terminate the course. The other assistant principal started talking, stating that I should keep going with the course in case I failed a subject. I felt a bit offended at his lack of belief for me. I backed myself to pass those subjects and he started throwing in 'what if' scenarios. *What if you fail a subject? What if you get sick again? What if something happens that you cannot complete the year?* His negativity and skepticism was rubbing off on me the wrong way. I wanted to press the mute button. This made me put up my boxing gloves and speak back fighting words. *Don't you worry about me. I am on track to pass. I will see this through.* His expression seemed to have a snarl, or it might just have been me perceiving it. I used this as ammunition to prove him wrong at the end of the year. I used it to add fuel to my fire. I would not allow him to be right. The other assistant principal, thankfully, backed me up and stated that I was doing well and was on track to pass, barring a major catastrophe. I walked away confident again that I would achieve the goal I had been striving for.

It was as if Doubt came back to try to shake me up to make me fall off my path. He was jealous of my friendship with God and the belief, faith and strength in which God had instilled in me. There was the episode of hives, the lack of enjoyment from the course, and now, the prospect of failing. I really hoped nothing else was going to be attempted to knock me off my goal. I felt puffed up after having to present my case and defend myself to the assistant principal. *I got this. I can do this. I will do this.* I spoke encouragement over myself to help me push through. I got rid of the dead weight with the course, and I was so close to my final term. I was ready to push forward; I did not want any more setbacks.

Virus.

I woke up with a painful feeling above my left eye. I moved to the mirror and saw three pimple-like spots. *I must be getting stressed because this is a bad pimple outbreak.* I began to try popping the pimples, but it was incredibly painful and I began to think that maybe these were too abnormal to be pimples. I drove to my local doctor to see what it might be. I began to get sharp, painful bursts every now and then, which added to my confusion. After waiting, I plopped myself into the doctor's office and I shared my concern of what was happening to my forehead. Before I could even finish, there was a very concerned expression on his face. He immediately stated that it was shingles. He hurried me to go to the emergency ward at the hospital, which was thirty minutes away. My eye began to swell up as if I had been king hit. I panicked and began driving to the hospital. No thought told me to contact my family, but to just drive myself straight there. I could still see, despite my swollen eye, but the pain bursts continually put me at risk while driving, as it took my attention away momentarily, like sharp knives stabbing my head. The adrenaline kicked in and I began speeding my way there. The day had gone from one to one hundred quickly. As I was driving, I saw my swollen eye in the mirror and it scared me. I muttered a prayer to God. *God, you have taken my hearing, I will not let you take my sight away.* I prayed with such conviction because fear of the added limitation to my deafness was suffocating.

I was speeding through, as the thought of getting there quicker was a priority for me. I sped past a speed camera and, thankfully, no light flashed. In a hurry, I finally arrived at the emergency ward and because of the potential contagion of my condition; the nurses scuttled me into a very dark room. I explained the situation, filled in the form, and shared my background of bone marrow transplant. Throughout these conversations, the forehead pain continued to pulsate. A nurse noticed my swollen and bloated eye; communicating an apprehensive expression. She asked if I could see. *I can see you just fine, as if I didn't have a swollen eye.* She nodded her head unconvincingly. I was left to myself, as they gave me painkillers. Half an hour later, the same nurse walked in and asked the same question: *Can you see me?* I responded with the exact same answer. She continued to be unconvinced, as if she was expecting me to lose my eyesight. I was a little bothered. Again, she left me alone, until thirty minutes after. She asked the same question and I responded the same way. I was becoming rather annoyed, for she did not believe me.

She decided to put me to the test. At the end of the room, there was an eye test sheet with all the letters, arranged from big to small. I sat upright and stated all the letters on the sheet... from top to bottom. Biggest to smallest. I had never correctly analysed all the letters before. I was quite surprised, but no more surprised than my nurse. She became convinced and believed that I could actually see. After a three hour stay, they patched up my shingles, assigned me some antibiotics to assist in my recovery and told me to rest until I was healthy again. My parents picked me up and I was absolutely exhausted. Sleep was all I wanted. I crashed on the couch and barely stayed awake for more than ten minutes. Everything was put on hold while I recovered. I worried about my schooling, but I knew I could miss a few days, for I had been diligent in my attendance so far. My priority was to get better as quick as possible. I slept the next few days away until my body began to click into gear and demanded to be up and moving. Eventually, the scabbing of the shingles began to fall away and I could pick it off. A scarring developed where it used to reside. My eye began to shrink back to normality.

My energy slowly came back. Soon, I was able to resume my schooling commitments, with an obvious reminder of what just occurred with the scarring above my eyes. More battle scars. More victories. I was thankful that I had overcome a setback once again and could continue to finish the work I had started. I did not take the privilege lightly. As I shared with someone what happened, she became shocked and told me that someone got the exact same thing I did, in the exact spot, and she lost her eyesight. Due to the inflammation of the virus, it burnt off the nerve endings within her eyes. It hit me, remembering the nurse's disbelief in my claim to sight. I realized that I probably should have lost my eyesight as a result. In that moment, I felt a warm hand over my shoulder and saw that God was smiling towards me. I thanked him for his protection and for hearing my prayer not to lose my sight. God had my back once again. Every setback had been a set up for God to do something greater. I drew strength from this thought and continued to move forward with greater belief than before.

Declaration.

I encountered a friend whom I had not seen since my hospital stay. He marvelled at the opportunity to see me again and that I was up and about. As we caught up, he shared something profound about my own Dad. *James, I will never forget what your dad said to me when he told me how ill you were. He was so defiant and demanded the word of God be true. He demanded that there was no way you would be lost to him, as Jesus said he would not make us go through more than we could bear. And with that, God would save you. This made me pray so much for your dad and you.* I was overwhelmed with the thought of this about my Dad; I became so proud of him. Never have I felt someone so strongly advocate for me and back me up. Never have I felt so loved before. It was out of his love that Dad wanted to declare strongly that I would not lose. I began to understand why Dad had been such a powerful voice into my battle and my challenges. I had a Dad who was determined not to lose me and he carried that mindset from the start to the end, not allowing any negativity or doubt come to my mind. From my anaphylactic attack, being in ICU, to my recovery timeline, my schooling future, my bout with hives and attack of shingles, he stood firm in faith. Every word he spoke into those situations enabled me to fight through with strength. It is amazing how thoughts do matter when it comes to facing battles. Dad spoke in faith and I spoke in increasing faith. These two strong stances allowed no space for failure and warranted God to reward the faith and the conviction we had. Thoughts count! I thank the friend who shared the story and became encouraged further.

Magnitude.

Examinations were coming and I wanted to wind down. I looked for a movie to watch and I decided on *My Sister's Keeper*. I had no idea what it was about and it turned out to be a family who has a daughter/sister going through cancer. It was an interesting movie to watch, since it was the first movie I watched about cancer since going through my own battle of it. As I watched the movie alone, the themes of setbacks, survival and death hit me. It hit me hard, moving me to tears. *This could have been my* tears. The film shows the impact one person's sickness can have on the family. The mother quits her job, the parents' marriage is strained due to the focus being on the sick daughter. The older brother is getting up to trouble because of the lack of attention, while the younger sister is born purely to keep the sick sister alive through compatible blood and platelet donations. The main reason I became a sobbing and weeping mess is when the daughter knows she is about to die. I spent the last thirty minutes of the movie saying *this could have been me*. I could not help placing myself in her situation and ponder the effects it could have had on my family and onwards. I never once thought I would not make it. *How would I respond? How would I feel?*

The magnitude and immensity of what I had overcome hit me with a ton of bricks. I never realized the devastation cancer could cause because I was so caught up in the middle of the battle that I used every ounce of focus and strength to push myself through. God's comforting assurance and affirmation of his promises cloaked me throughout the storm that I never looked the other way. I thank God for giving me a new lease on life. I look at all the new experiences, new friendships and new opportunities I had gained in the past eight months. *I could have easily missed this*. In that moment, I had never felt so important, so significant… so valued! The enormity of the battle hit me. The thought humbled me: I have overcome something massive. The potential damage of cancer was so huge, but I won! My family won! God won! I continued to thank God for my second chance. I thanked Dad for being so adamant that I would not be taken away from him, as it would be unbearable for him. I thank everyone else for their prayers, the time they put in for me, as it did make a difference. In my sobbing mess, it was probably the first real reflection I had done during my battle and it was a powerful reflection. God began to share with me, *every person in life that you encounter is valuable. Sometimes you get caught up in going through the motions; participating in the logistics of life and forget to invest quality time with people around you. You all have something to offer people and people all have something to offer you. Relationships are powerful. Relationships are why I created you so I can be with you, you can be with me, and you can all be with each other. Do not forget this.* I am able to see people through the eyes of God as he imparts his treasured thoughts about his creation. After crying for an hour, I caught my breath and thanked God for the powerful realization of what I had gone through and the value of people. I pray that I never forget this onwards.

Holidays.

September 2011. The holidays before exams had arrived. It was a strange sensation. I have come this far, yet this mountain was the last challenge I needed in order to tick off all my goals that I established while I was sick. It was a fantastic thought, knowing these exams are the final exams I would ever do in high school. I was so close, yet so far, as my brain was already tired of schoolwork and I only had an ounce of motivation left. Part of me wanted to simply do the least possible to pass, but another part wanted me to do my absolute best so I could be proud of my efforts. The classes were wrapping up and I was tired of classes because my brain had possibly overloaded in its power due to the big workload so soon after being in hospital. Although, God kept refreshing me and my goal kept me focused and in tune to the task. It was a very contradicting approach.

Dinner.

As the classes wrapped up, there was a Valedictorian Dinner to celebrate the year of schooling before Examinations. I put forward a request to do a speech to express my sincere thanks and deep gratitude to the support given by the staff, teachers and students. The school granted me permission to speak towards the end of the night. It was exciting and humbling to be given the opportunity. These people did not comprehend the value their support had brought to me. With no support, there was a lack of motivation and I would not have been able to be standing in that place, ready to finish my school after exams. After sweating nerves, it became time to deliver the speech. I shared the struggles of battling cancer and the challenge of going back to school. This challenge was met by the unwavering support of all the people in the room. I singled out specific people who had moments where they encouraged me and gave me confidence to continue. I finished off with an urge to remember that we can always support each other, love each other and urge each other onwards to greater things. There was a rousing applause by everyone that had played a small but significant part in my personal challenge. I never fought this battle alone. God used this moment to share a picture of the people I was impacting through my story, and the people who were impacting me as I journeyed through life. This is a beautiful aspect of life to be aware of and appreciated.

Practice.

With the pre-celebrations over and the final holidays embarking before exams, there was only one more challenge between me and my final goal of completing school: finishing examinations successfully. I worked out that I am not the most studious student, but also not the least. I did like discovering and learning. I needed to find out the best way for me to do something in order to position myself to succeed. I stared at my blank white bedroom wall, trying to figure out how. Having to open each book and study was not the best way for me to go about it motivation wise. Something clicked in my mind: *What if there is a way to keep every book open?* This lead me to the bright idea of writing all the relevant information for each subject on mammoth-sized paper and hanging it up on the bare wall. I sat there, going through all my notes and transferring it onto the paper. In the process, I was able to be refreshed with my study notes. I hung it up on my wall and took a step back, marvelling at my project. All I had to do now was simply walk it and reflect on these notes. It was a visual experience as well as a mental lesson. It certainly helped me avoid having to push myself to open my textbooks and revise for hours on end. Throughout the holidays, I had a few practice exams to gain traction for the real deal, to find a rhythm and get feedback on incorrect answers. One by one, I knocked off the practice exams and the revision tasks set by the teacher. I was ready to knock off this mountain and stand atop in victory.

Examinations.

October 2011. First up was my three-hour English exam. It was purely based on writing, creativity and techniques. I dreaded it because I knew I had to push through mentally for a full three-hour block, but I was ready to go for it. I had nothing to lose. I had worked hard to get to this point. I had trusted God and I was inching very close to finishing the school year in one year as I boldly spoke I would do—despite all the doubt from others and the challenges I faced. Surely this seemed minimal compared to what had occurred for the past two years. *This is the final English exam you have to do. Ever.* I gave myself a pep-talk and start knocking it out. As I went on, my fingers started aching from the constant writing. To my shock, I saw a groove developing in my finger where my pen was pressing hard against. *Just push through James, push through.* I was aware of the race against the clock, but making progress. By the time I completed the final sentence of my second essay, the time was up. One down, four to go.

Next one was Maths. An hour and a half is easy compared to the three-hour English Exam. I grew in confidence, feeling I had done the hardest one already. Knowing Maths was my strength, I gave it my best crack and walked away knowing I had given it my best. Up next was Media, just need to know my Media terms and analysis. I felt the full backing of my revision and studies. Completed. Only two left. Another Math Exam, except this one was even easier due to being a multiple-choice exam. I knocked it down and I only had one left. Business Management. Just needed to knuckle down on the terminology and case study issues. This was it. The final work I had to do and I was done. I could not begin to comprehend the idea that I was about to finish high school education forever. I was getting ahead of myself and reeled it back in quickly. *Focus James, Focus!*

Final.

I walked into the schoolroom for my final examination. It was a strange time for an exam, 4.00 p.m. compared to the others being early morning. There was a refreshing scent in the air. I was so close I could feel it; I could taste it. I was walking out of here a free man. I shook my focus back into the room. Teacher called for the exam to start and I was furiously scribbling away. Each word I did was one word I would never do again. I was excited as each page was completed. After the final case study. I put down my pen, handed in my exam and walked out. A smile was brimming on my face. Nothing was on my mind. A weight was not felt on my shoulders for the first time in a long time. No worries nor anxiety existed in my mind. *I did it. I have finished.* I said nothing to no one, instead stepping into my car and driving away. I turned up the music and rolled down the window. I simply wanted to soak in this feeling. It was accomplishment, freedom, joy, gratitude and peace meshed all at once. The satisfaction of victory soaked into me like a warm bubble bath. The fulfilment of my partnership with God generated a sense of pride. This could not be achieved without God's hand and work in my life, nor would it have been completed if I did not press in full of faith.

I felt the intimacy of God as I reflected on this. *Thank you, God. Thank you so much. We did it.* I reflect on the relationship that has developed with God. *You have never let me down. Only built me up and onwards. I gave you a chance when I gave you my life and you have grabbed it with both hands.* Appreciation swelled up within me; a tear of joy streamed down my cheek. So many people had prayed, supported and shared their love for me during this crazy season and none of it has been wasted. *All of it is propelling me closer to you God, your plan for me, and to the greatest victory I have achieved so far today; fighting my battles in stronger faith with you. I am never turning away from you God. Not after all you have done.* My faith became cement in stone, never to be removed.

Result.

December 16th, 2011. The date of the release of results finally arrived. I woke up and frantically checked how to find out. There was a sense of peace, knowing I only needed to pass, but a competitive side in me wanted to know how I did. After a few technology issues, I eventually discovered the score. It sat in front of me. I was blown away. With the understanding of the accumulation of hardship I faced, the challenges I endured, and not having the backing of the fifth subject to help me, pride hit me. It was there in its finality. Nothing could take it away from me. Whatever happened now, I do not have to go back to high school again. My final goal has been checked off. I was back at school, playing basketball, participating in the school sports tradition and had a speedy recovery. Everything I spoke in faith, set into motion, had come to a completion.

I arrived back at school to pick up the hard copy of my report. I bumped into the Assistant Principal, who had been giving me a hard time all year, not showing an ounce of support; expecting me to fail or become sick again. He had a coffee mug in his hand, leaning onto the doorframe. A smug smile rubbed on his face. *Did you pass? Are you happy with your score?* He pestered me for an answer. I smiled and nodded my head. Building up the suspense, I held my tongue for a moment. I emphatically shared my score. On his face, a smile turned into shock. It was priceless. He was absolutely gobsmacked and speechless. It felt like I gave him an uppercut to the face. It was a pleasure, knowing that he could not comprehend the simple fact that I had pushed through what I endured and exceeded the bold statements I made at the start of the year, mixing it with the great score I finished with. I walked away, leaving him in his shocked state. Through God, anything is possible.

▰▰▰ EPILOGUE.

July 2018. I stand here today, over seven years after my treatment, fully healed. I am past the remission stage, which means that I am at my lowest risk of relapsing. God is faithful to his promise that I will never receive chemotherapy again. This chapter in my life is closed. I now carry this testimony as a story that reminds me of how amazing God is when it comes to walking with me in my battles. The last seven years since my treatment has provided me with many different seasons, each with their own unique set of challenges—financially, relationally, physically, emotionally, mentally and spiritually. The same principle remains: in each battle, God is helping me as I surrender to God and hand over my battles.

My fight against cancer has impacted my relationship with God, my character and my outlook on life positively. It might have been a painful journey, but it is a beautiful scar that has moulded me as a man and as the man God wants me to become. It is exciting to see what more God has for me in the future.

I have people questioning my beliefs in God when it comes to this situation. People often attempt to convince me that God doesn't have anything to do with my battle and recovery. Rather, it is the fact that it is due to the amazing medical team, science and my inner strength that drove me to a great recovery. I am not taking any credit away from the people who work at the hospital; the many hours they have put in to study, research and sharpen their craft as doctors and nurses. I am always thankful for their hard work that leads to them being of great support in giving me a new lease in life. In saying so, I know that, without God, I do not make it out of this battle. There are too many signs for it to be ignored. There is the first moment of surrendering it over to God and holding onto his everlasting hope that gave me something foundational and firm to stand upon.

There is the moment where he clogs up my throat to ensure I could not take my sleeping pills. There is the moment he gave me rest from my illness when I needed it. There is the miracle of me not losing my sight when I had shingles strike the nerve-endings of my eye. Along with this, he sustains me throughout and follows through the revelation he handed to me in 2007, which is *to have a life-inspiring story that will change people's lives.* I have seen and experienced too much for me to deny that God is real. There is absolutely no turning back for me for my faith is cemented in conviction. This situation refined my faith from doubting God to absolutely knowing with one hundred percent conviction that God is real and alive today! It all began with me giving God a chance to do something in my life as I get to know him. Brick by brick, he built up my faith in him, to the point I had to stand in the house and fight for my faith as it is put to the test through the challenges. This is what the fight of faith is.

██████ RESOURCE.

The Testimony I spoke on a Men's night in Feb 2011

I want this story to encourage you to hand over your situation or problem to our God. We are all different. We all have different problems but the same principle remains - we all have problems. Along with that, we serve the same God. So when you go home tonight, or whenever you get the chance, I want you to hand over whatever situation you are in to God and pray like a warrior.

But there are conditions! Once you give it to God, you are to leave it to him. You should not wait around until one little thing goes wrong and then take it away from him and try deal with it yourself again. You are pretty much digging yourself a bigger hole. It will show that you have no trust in God, no faith, no confidence in God. The whole purpose of hardships is to strengthen and define you and your relationship with God.

So whatever hardship you are facing in life, let us trust God to handle it and work through it with him. As we can become Godly people, people of faith, people of conviction and people of strength, the amount of people that will be inspired by your courage and faith will be innumerable. God is waiting and willing. All he is waiting for is you to be willing to trust in him. Take that step of faith and crazy good things are going to happen in your life and God's blessing will overflow.

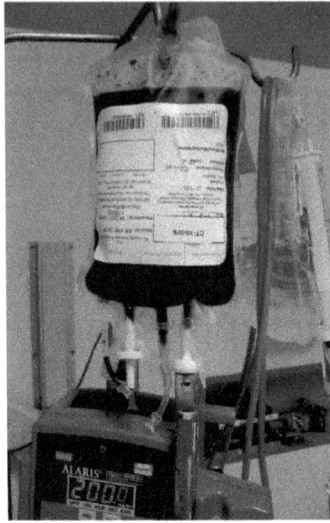

The bone marrow that was donated from a French woman
who was compatible for my bone marrow

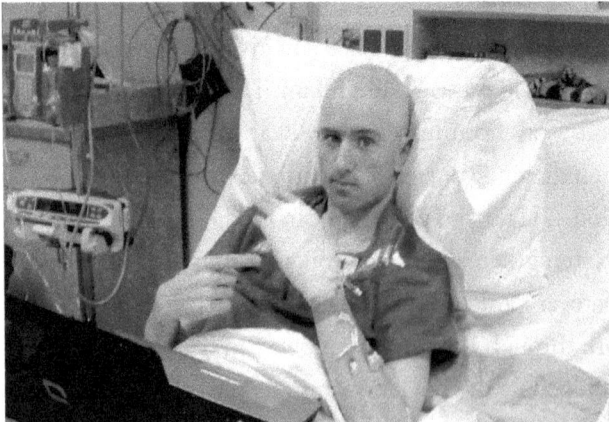

A bandaged hand after receiving the entire bone marrow transplant through
hand as well as a swollen mouth as after effects of anaphylactic attack

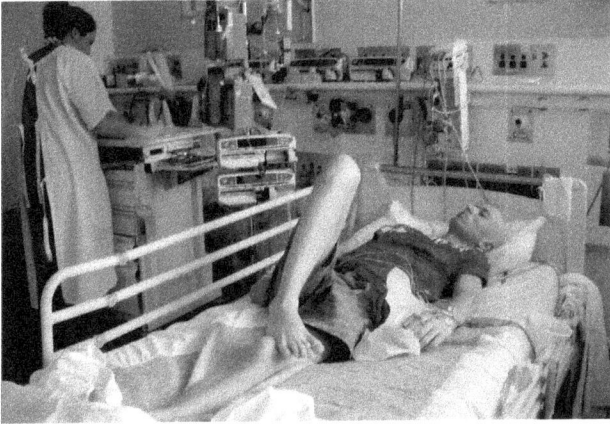

The dreary morning after the anaphylactic attack while also having to
fast for the day to prepare for surgery to have a new Hickman line

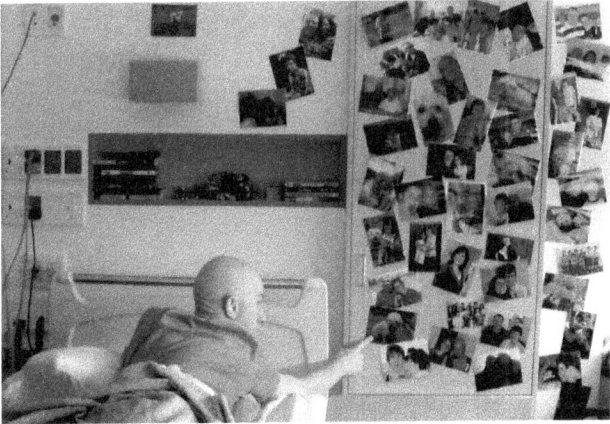

My personal photo collection to feel support from those whom
I love and adore while in isolation for six months.

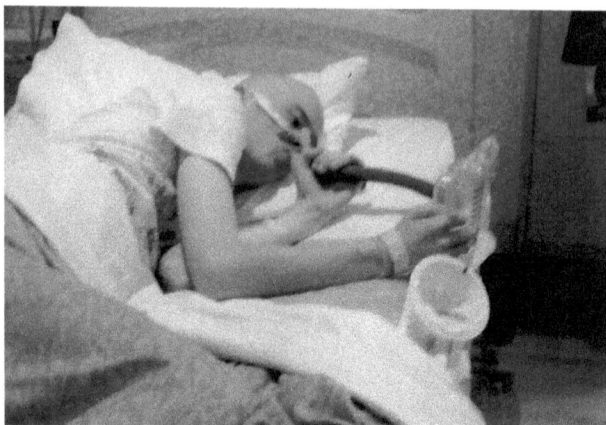

The horrible and demanding breathing exercises I had to endure
to build up my lung capacity after suffering pneumonia.

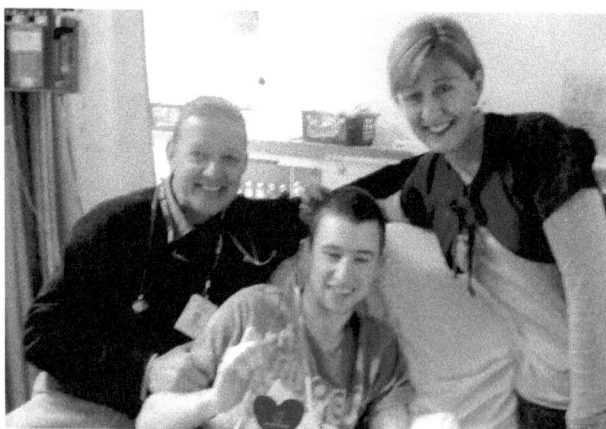

Dr Peter and Katie, who looked after me in my pre-diagnosis, handing over the
Monash Inspirational Award which was a great reminder of the promise God gave me

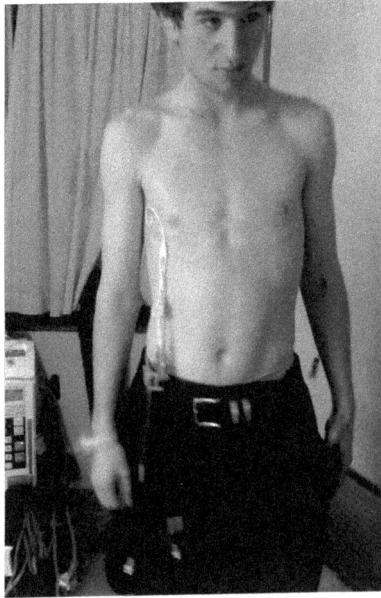

The Hickman Line inserted under arms to provide ease for transfusions of blood, platelets, chemo, transplant, and fluids

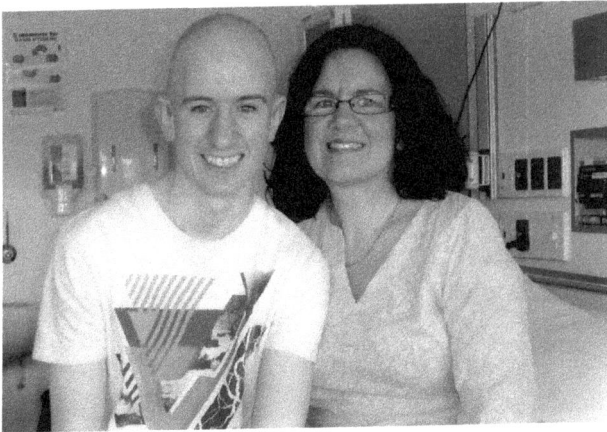

My mother and I on our first day of my isolation period preparing for second round of chemotherapy

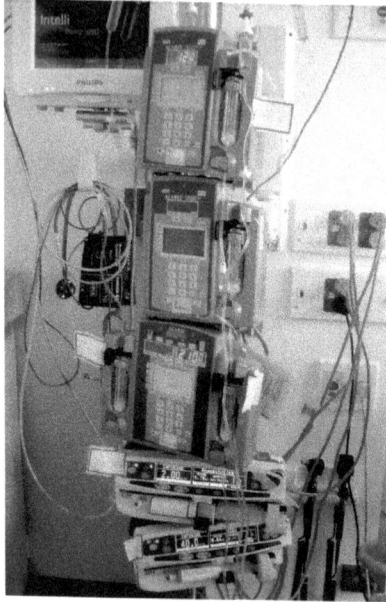

My personal patient monitor that was a little overloaded with equipment and cables! Led me to the horrid accident one night.

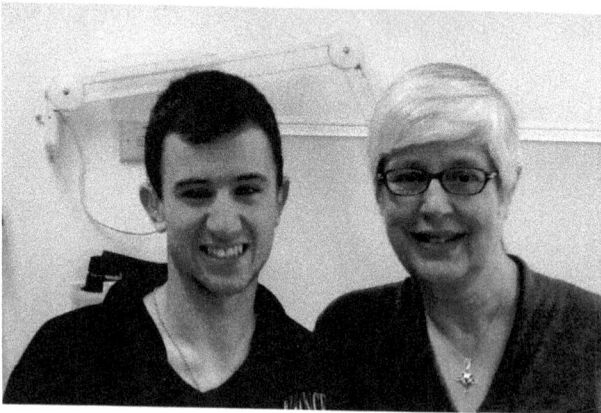

The wonderful Dr Karin, who was fantastic in looking after, and challenging me in all aspects of my health and recovery.